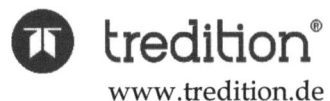

www.tredition.de

AF190278

Veronika Esslinger

The script of your Life

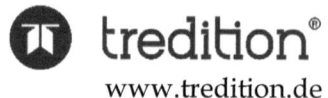

www.tredition.de

© 2019 Veronika Esslinger

Publishing Company & Print: tredition GmbH, Halenreie 40-44
22359 Hamburg

ISBN
Paperback: 978-3-7497-3712-3
Hardcover: 978-3-7497-3713-0
e-Book: 978-3-7497-3714-7

Imprint:

Author: Veronika Esslinger
Design and Co-Author:
MS Design, Melanie Stadelbauer
Bloggerherz, Christian Gera

The work including its parts is protected by copyright. Any use
is prohibited without the consent of the publisher and the
author. This applies in particular to electronic or other
duplication, translation, distribution and public disclosure.

Think carefully about what you're wishing for and work hard to make your dreams come true. I'm thankful to my parents & friends, for being by my side through all ups and downs and for allowing me to live my dreams.

Good friends listen to your story; true friends help you write it.

Thanks to Karin Seven, actress & coach from Berlin, for your support and your unwavering faith in me.

Thanks to Anna Russo, Make-Up-Artist from Los Angeles, for your inspiration & friendship.

Table of contents

Prolog

Where do I begin? How could I reveal my inner thoughts to the outside? How do I write my book and tell my very own story? I observe a butterfly flap its wings, time stands still. With closed eyes, I sit on a park bench in late summer. Right in the center of Berlin. The wind gently touches my skin, I can feel goosebumps on my arms and a chilly breeze clears my mind …

"WHATEVER YOU CAN DO OR DREAM YOU CAN; BEGIN IT."

-JOHANN WOLFGANG VON GOETHE

I had only just read this sentence on a wall in the park. They touched my soul deep inside. At first, I was startled like a young deer when I discovered these words, but then I recognized their depth; an abyss even. I needed to think things through and I needed to decide which path I was going to take in my life. Here and now. On this park bench in late summer. The time was there to take a look back and put the puzzle pieces together. Like a butterfly, my thoughts flew off and unfolded my previous life before me ….

Emma's life has never been a piece of cake. Even when she was still young, she had to prove herself to her family and the people around her. She always stood in her sister's shadow.

But Emma found a way, her very own way in fact, to live out her potential and her passion. A couple of years later, she even founded her own company and kept overcoming any obstacles standing in her way. She gained confidence and strength and mastered all hurdles. Setbacks and low blows couldn't stop her. All of this – especially the failures - are what makes or breaks a person at the end of the day.

But what happened to her? Where were all the glory and the glamour? The applause? She could have all of that. But did she even still want it? She was sad and torn apart inside, but she had a clear mind and she was focused. But why did she feel this way now?

Emma was a successful business woman with two beauty salons. She was living in Berlin, in a beautiful apartment in the green... Just like she had always dreamed of, but deep inside she was still looking for her true purpose.

Something was missing. She looked at her life in some kind of bird's-eye view. The higher she flew, the smaller she felt. An abyss opened in front of the park bench she was sitting on.

Should she jump? Should she rather stay? Which path should she choose? ...What was it that tore her apart inside?

She was regularly booked as a choreographer and dancer. That was her passion, her hobby, her muse. She was just about to make a break-through as an actress as well.

But then there was this one single encounter that changed her life en-tirely. Matthews, an actor from Hollywood.

A dangerous amour, marked by love, suffering and intrigues. Be careful what you wish for, because it might come true.

The Script of your Life is a story with depth, heartache and tragedy.

... Which path would Emma choose?

Which role in life would she take on?

Go on a journey of life in "the City of Angels" affected by drama, rumors and dangerous love affairs... but especially with the knowledge that dreams come true despite all obstacles in life.

"If you can dream it, you can do it!" (Walt Disney)

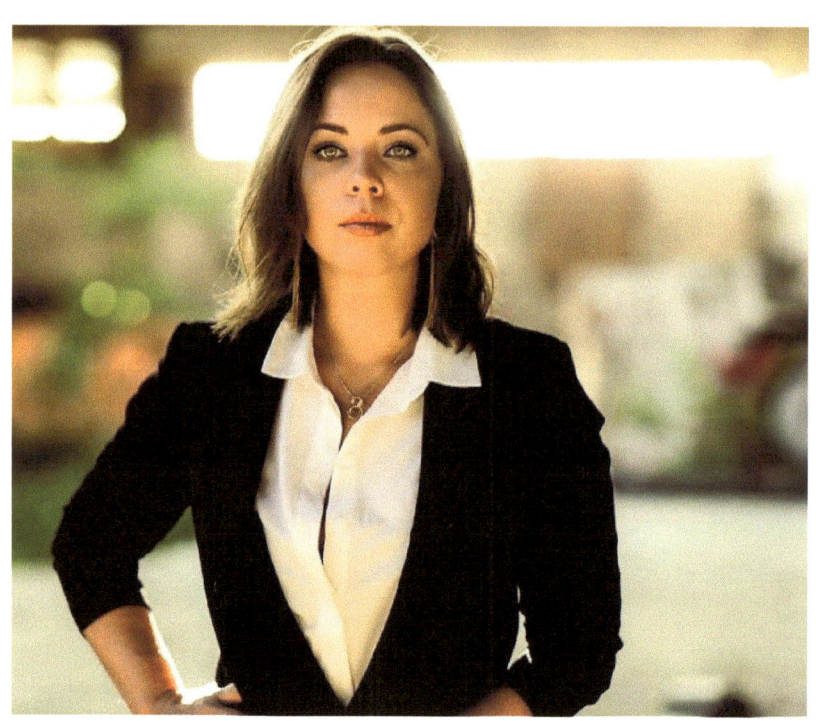

V Esslinger

New beginning and dreams

My new life situation was a challenge. In this year, I had split up with my ex-fiancé. Not that he minded; he just moved on with the next woman in the house that we had lived in together.

When I moved out of the house this summer, I was pretty sure my world would crumble. I had to look for a new place to stay. Fortunately, I had good friends and so I could crash at my friends' place in Zürich for three weeks. She tried to comfort me and lovingly took care of me. "Forget about Richard" Vanessa said every day. But that was easy for her to say. Our wedding was set already. Meanwhile, with the help of a real estate agent I befriended, a client in my beauty salon, I searched for a new apartment.

Vanessa asked me to not stay home all day and drown myself in self-pity: Zürich was right outside the door! She was working as a barkeeper in a popular scene bar right in the center of Zürich.

"Come with me, forget about Richard!" she demanded.

Eventually, I gave in to her demands with a heavy heart. Prettied up, yet quite empty inside still, we went to the lounge bar.

I didn't really feel like dealing with a big crowd of people. Vanessa was quite busy herself. So, I sat down at the bar counter where, luckily, there weren't too many people. Vanessa came by right away and poured a glass of Rosé champagne for me. Was there even anything for me to celebrate? According to Vanessa, I did, but according to myself, I did not. I was still deeply hurt...

A man in his forties took a seat next to me. I could feel his glance on me; he must have liked what he saw. I could feel this chemistry between us right away.

He talked to me in English without any accent. His pronunciation was as perfect as I had last heard it in Los Angeles when I visited the city...

I told him about my beauty salon and that I was also working as a professional dancer/choreographer on the side. And he actually did come from Los Angeles and worked as a producer in Hollywood.

Incredible!... was my first thought, and obviously, any man could tell you the same, if he was trying to hookup. But my guts told me he was indeed a nice and honest guy from Los Angeles. Crazy how life goes sometimes and how fate sometimes brings people together in the most exceptional situations. Especially when you don't expect it.

It was a great evening which slowly drew to an end. In the end, we exchanged numbers.

Right away, I began doing some research regarding my new acquaintance; highly amused and grinning, Vanessa just shook her head. "Sweetie, do you seriously think this guy is for real? And what then? Do you think, Bill is just going to give you a role in one of his movies and then you're becoming famous?"

"I mean, duh!" I said laughing.

As it turned out in the end, he really didn't lie. Vanessa snapped my phone out of my hand and stared at the online results and pictures just as dumbfounded.

She stopped the car, turned around towards me and grabbed my shoulder with a dead serious expression on her face:

"Imagine this was your breakthrough! That would be incredible" euphoric and with all kinds of Hollywood dreams in our luggage, we drove towards the last sunrays of the day...

When my phone rang the next morning, I was shocked and so excited at the same time – it was Bill the Hollywood producer. Of course, I didn't want to show how nervous I was. I was so excited I barely could get a word out of my mouth.

Fortunately, Bill was a bit more experienced than me and got straight to the point. "Hi, it's me, Bill. I wanna say thanks for the great evening yesterday at the Lounge bar, it was really nice to meet you."

I managed to stay calm despite the excitement about his call, as the famous caller rather quickly clouded my euphoria about seeing him again soon:

Since the filming for his new movie started soon, he had to leave that night and go back to LA. I was so sad about this. Bill might have noticed at the other end.

"When you come to Los Angeles, let`s meet for a coffee! I'll show you the City of Angels. Let's stay in touch!"

I wanted to keep in contact. I felt a strong connection to him. Even if the wounds of my breakup were still fresh. I wanted to get out, away from here. And I firmly believed that we would meet soon again...

It was a rainy afternoon in November, I was visiting Zurich again and met friends at an art exhibition. There were a lot of people but I separated myself from the crowd to enjoy the art in peace.

I stopped in front of a Monet; the picture fascinated me.

To my right, I noticed an attractive, dark-haired man in elegant clothes. He was focused on the same picture as I was. He looked to the left when our eyes met.

We smiled at each other and then looked back at the art.

"Hi, I'm Matthews!" he said surprised.

"Hello, my name is Emma!" - ... "beautiful art exhibition, wouldn't you agree, Emma?"

... I nodded reservedly and didn't really show any interest in Matthews, yet he kept going.

Matthews, a tall, lean and imposing man with such a breath-taking aura – at least to me – who was particularly good at being mysterious... we talked in a way that made me forget anything around me.

"Emma, would you be interested in having a little appetizer with me at the bar?" He expressed himself according to his appearance. "I'd like that" I replied.

Arriving at the bar, Matthews showed genuine interest in my life; I told him about my career. Then I got curious myself and wanted to hear more of his own story.

"I'm an actor and I live in Los Angeles; I am just here for a visit…"

I couldn't believe it; once again I met someone from Los Angeles; in Zurich, as well. Could there even be coincidences like these in life? This city seemed to magically attract me somehow.

"Wow, color me impressed!" "No, what you are doing is impressing" Matthews countered. We smiled and right away, there was this magic surrounding us.

Do you know these kinds of evenings and nights that pass in slow motion, where you forget anything around you?

We turned night to day by dancing through the bars and clubs of the city. I forgot about Richard.

Even if nobody said it out loud, we both knew there was something special between us. We already planned a second meeting which was supposed to take place in Paris…

Paris

I loved this city. Even more I loved the thought of seeing Matthews again the next day!

Months passed after our first meeting and the desire to see him again took over me. I felt taken back to when I was 17, to my time as a teenager!

Matthews managed to get us two tickets for the Moulin Rouge Show, a table with the perfect view at the stage. I was more than happy. I could feel a tingling in my entire body...

Slowly, the weight of my past and my breakup with Richard; my entire old life so to say, was lifted off my shoulders.

Matthews seemed to have noticed that as well as he was excited about how much I could let my guard down around him.

Moulin Rouge, here we go...

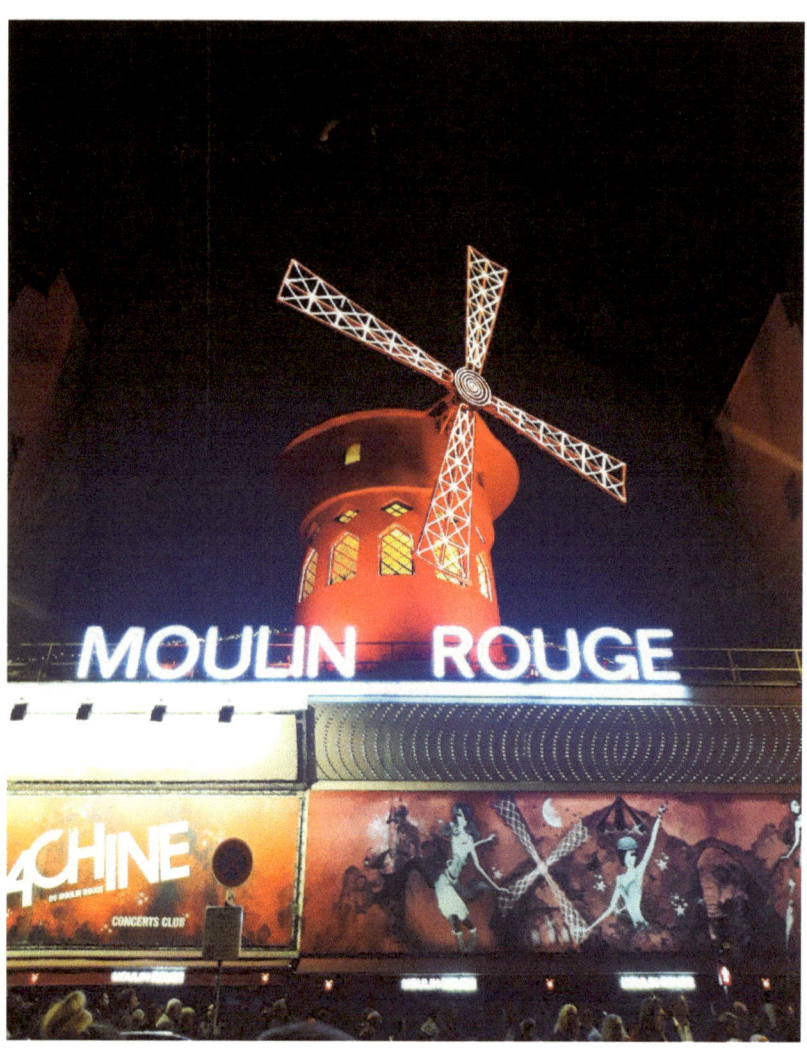

But before it could get there, I traveled ahead to meet my aunt. She lived in Paris, not far away from the Moulin Rouge and I had a key to her apartment. She was going to be in her apartment to welcome me the next day.

As a fashion designer, she was traveling the world a lot and I was really looking forward to seeing her again. She turned into a typical Parisian lady. Always dressed well, one package of cigarettes a day, sometimes more. Her perfect French sounded so elegant and the way she expressed herself was always on point. She knew the Parisian fashion scene which I appreciated a lot and she never was at a loss for words.

I was so excited, what should I wear? Which pair of shoes would work, if I picked a dress? Or rather pants with a fitting blouse? No, rather a dress.

"I'd grab the little black dress, if I was you!" auntie said, to make it easier for me to decide – and smoked one of her long cigarettes.

The bright red lipstick she wore emphasized her elegant, chic look combined with her widely-cut coat and the fitting hat.

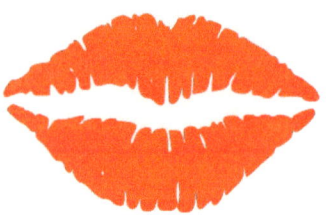

Her updo hairstyle let a few strands of her silver hair shine through beneath the wide brim of her hat. I liked her purposely elegant style. "Come here, I'll style your hair. A light wave perhaps, so you don't appear so strict?"

I let her decide and trusted her blindly, since she was a style icon to me anyways. Two hours left before the show started. I did decide for the little black dress, my hair was done in a gentle wave that playfully covered a part of my face. Smokey Eyes, but not too overdone and a hint of red lipstick. The black and gray glitter High heels rounded off the outfit. The Chanel perfume gave a subtle erotic hint that I wanted to achieve.

After the styling, I was so nervous that my aunt poured me another glass of Rosé champagne.

"Here's to a great evening!" she said and raised her glass as well. ... I really had to visit her more often, I thought to myself....

The noble penthouse apartment of my aunt was indeed quite impressive! Its location rounded off the atmosphere well. I loved Paris and its diversity and the individuality of the people. Just the smell which was ever-present in the little streets of Paris. A mixture of smoke, perfume, creativity and danger! But that was what made the city so exciting.

The vibration of my phone brought me back to reality.

"Well? Is it Matthews" The suggestive grin on my auntie's face said it all.

"Yes, indeed. He only just arrived. You can't even imagine how nervous I am!" Quickly, I put on my beige coat on top of my little black dress...

It was only 10 minutes walking distance to the Moulin Rouge. But walking there seemed to take an eternity. It was a chilly evening in January. Despite the bad weather, a lot of people were sitting outside the cafés to the sides of the Parisian streets.

With every step I made, I felt more and more nervous.

There was already a huge crowd gathering in front of the gates to the famous Varietés. And then I saw him. His elegant appearance almost reminded me of "Joe Black"... He wore a black suit, a white shirt underneath and a black bow tie. A Chanel scarf in beige rounded off his style.

There was a smile on his face when he saw me. I couldn't believe it. It was him indeed! Matthews! And he looked so good!

Nervously, I kept forcing myself to calm down as I walked towards him. My aunt sure knew what she was doing when she poured me the champagne. It didn't miss its effect.

"Hi!" we said at the same time. He gave me a warm hug that I would have liked to drown in. "Hi" I said again and smiled. "That's a long line, I hope you're going to enjoy the show. I've seen it once before and the performance was amazing, such an artistic pleasure!"

The crowd slowly moved towards the entrance. I could feel the sparks flying between Matthews and me.

"Welcome to the Moulin Rouge, please enjoy the show!" the man at the entrance said. There were well-dressed and highly excited people all around us. The atmosphere was exciting itself and inspiring at the same time.

"If you'd like to, we could go to a restaurant afterwards" Matthews said. "I know some secret gems around here!" Of course, we could. Happiness was flowing through my entire body as I couldn't believe those words. "Yes, I'd love that!"

Even when his phone rang, the tingling in my stomach didn't stop. He answered his phone and greeted the person on the other end in his perfect English without any accent.

His manly, demanding tone made my body shudder. "I'm glad to hear from you…!" Who was he talking to? His agency perhaps? I didn't know! What could have been this important that they had to call him on a Saturday night?

"…For real? I thought the script was amazing…! Also, the female role is the perfect counterpart to my male role! When do they start shooting? On Tuesday?

…Could you please book a good flight to LA for me? …"

When he hung up the phone, sadness took over me. We only just saw each other again after such a long period of time. And now he had to leave again?

"I'm so sorry, I just got a call from my agency. As you might have heard, I have to fly back to Los Angeles tomorrow, very early in the morning! I applied for a role in a movie and honestly didn't expect anymore that the producer would pick me. It's a drama, you're going to like it. You definitely have to watch the movie!"

"Wow, congratulation, I'm so happy for you!" I tried to hide my disappointment.

We only barely sat down at the table when a waiter came by with a bottle of champagne. It was perfect! The show started but I had my eyes on Matthews!

"Cheers, to a great evening!" he said raising his glass of champagne. We watched the show. It was fantastic and an artistic pleasure indeed! Matthews hadn't promised too much! The show kept getting better. The show kept getting better and better. In one moment, twenty women were dancing, when one of them jumped into a pool in the middle, which suddenly floated up out of the ground. A pool full of snakes. It was amazing to see how she was playing with so many snakes but still managed to move so gracefully.

As we strolled to the restaurant on the Champs-Élysées, I could feel the fire for him rising more and more inside of me. Somewhere in the back of my head there was still this fear of getting hurt, which certainly slowed down even greater emotions inside of me. Or maybe that was just a good human defense mechanism. Either way, I was glad that I could still let my guard down. I couldn't control my feelings for Matthews anyways - they overwhelmed and somehow sparked an endless fire inside of me ...

Like a true gentleman, Matthews held the door to the restaurant open for me. It was a small but very fancy and cozy restaurant with French music playing in the background. We ate and talked about our first meeting, what projects he was working on and about his goals. We excitedly talked about all the things in our private and professional lives that we were passionate about.

The clock already struck midnight when we left the restaurant to go to the bar at the opposite side of the street for an appetizer. "Hey, Happy Birthday!" Matthews raised his glass.

„Here's to much more exciting time together!" I laughed. Suddenly, they played the song by Bradley Cooper & Lady Gaga and I fell head over heels in love with Matthews! I fell in love with a Hollywood actor! I forgot about anything else. I blocked out anything else around me.

"Sadly, I have to leave now. I wish I didn't have to, but I have to catch my flight to Los Angeles tomorrow."

"I know" I said with a sad voice. A hug from him made my heart beat faster once again. It was pounding like crazy. "Let's chat sometime, thanks for the nice evening. I appreciate staying in contact with you. You truly are something special!"

With these rather distanced words, he got in his taxi. Our taxis took us to different destinations. I drove back to my aunt while he went back to his hotel room. I was passing the night in review once again. But loneliness kept creeping up on me again. I sat there – holidays alone in Paris. Would I ever see him again?

When I looked at my phone, I saw I had eight missed calls from Matthews ... I tried to call him back but unfortunately, I couldn't reach him. A look at the clock suggested that he was probably still on the airplane.

I had fallen asleep on the couch with all my clothes on and needless to say, I wasn't really happy, no exciting eroticism that night...

When I walked to the big terrace after waking up and saw the Moulin Rouge, my phone rang ...

"Hi, how are you doing?" Matthews asked. It was nice to hear his voice. "Yes, everything's great. Where are you at the moment?"

"I had a little stop in Atlanta for an important business appointment. After that, I'll get back to Los Angeles. Last night was really nice."

"It reminded me of the movie Blue Valentine with Michelle Williams and Ryan Gosling. This scene when they had their first date and walked through the streets of the city. You should check it out, it's a movie about Dean and Cindy. They fell in love at first sight. Now, they have been married for years and are raising Cindy's daughter together. You need to see it!"

"I'll definitely do that!" I said. "One thing I'm wondering about though: you live in Los Angeles; There are so many gorgeous women and models. Why me?"

"You just blew my mind, the models in Los Angeles are so superficial. I'm not interested in them."

Wow, I thought to myself, was I dreaming? Now, I felt like one of those movie scenes and I was the female lead role. Matthews had me and my feelings completely wrapped around his finger.

We messaged each other every day. We always found something to talk about. I felt a kind of connection and kinship with him that words just couldn't describe.

"You're welcome to come to the Oscars in March with me!" Oh my god, I thought. Who wouldn't say yes to that? But unfortunately, I had to decline, because my salon was completely overbooked and I couldn't just leave my coworker alone.

I was in a taxi in Paris, on the way to the airport, back home to my now new apartment. To the place where everything reminded me of Richard again. I had to hold back my tears, there was the song "Porcelain" by Moby playing on the radio, and I just couldn't hold back my tears. I wanted to be with Matthews, but I couldn't. Was every love as fragile as porcelain? When would I finally be happy?

When I arrived at home, my everyday life caught up to me with clients and new choreographies for my dance jobs, for which I was regularly booked.

From time to time, however, this sadness and complete hopelessness overcame me again and again ... had I lost Matthews forever? I didn't understand how this could have happened to me once again. Did I always fall in love with the wrong men? I mean, one man, an actor from Hollywood, was supposed to have a different woman every day, but my feeling told me that it was different with him and that there was something special going on between us.

Or was I wrong? This man was thousands of miles away from me, I had never visited him at home and we didn't have a lot of time together either, which we would actually need in order to build up a long-term relationship.

All of this gradually made me feel more and more insecure. Weeks passed and I didn't hear anything from Matthews, should I forget him as soon as possible?

I had almost given up and tried to get over it when I received a message fromhim.

"Hi, sorry that I haven't gotten in touch for so long, I was so busy working on the movie. I hope you're fine?"

... and there it was, my expression lit up. I couldn't hold it back. "Hey, yes, I'm fine thank you!" I replied.

"I'm done filming so far, with my part in the movie!" How are you doing these days? I got to say that I'm still sorry that we had so little time in Paris and that I had to leave so fast. I would like to spend some more time with you. Anyways, I enjoyed a lot what we had. But I regret one thing – to not have kissed you!"

As soon as this sentence came out of his mouth, my feelings overwhelmed me! I didn't know how to respond to that. I was trapped and euphoric at once. Should I ultimately surrender to my feelings?

I decided to allow it ... with his words, he had finally cast a spell over me.

"I really enjoyed the time with you, but why didn't you just kiss me?" I replied.

He said: "Something like this takes time, it has to grow between two people, it is much more than a relationship between a man and a woman, it should be a friendship to begin with!"

This is what I had been wanting for years, his words touched my soul. That was this void in my heart that I couldn't fill before through any relationship! It struck me like a lightning bolt. Much more than that. What should I do now? Should I confess my feelings to Matthews?

In the following days I received advice from Vanessa. Of course, she told me I should follow my heart ....

"I can do it!" I told myself every day! I was going to do it!

We messaged each other back and forth every day as usual. When I said "Matthews, I fell in love!" he replied "With whom? Someone from work? That lucky guy."

"I fell in love with you!" I said and right away threw my phone into the next corner.

My God, what was I doing there? Was I crazy? So far, I (or we?) had only ever felt it - but never actually said it out loud. Not during the first meeting, not even at the art exhibition and the beautiful time in Zurich - and in Paris there was no time for it.

How could you even say that to a man before he said it first? And why was I overthinking it now?

I picked up my phone from the floor and saw a message from Matthews. I was afraid to open it! What would it say? Would he feel the same as I did?

"Wow, that's quite the surprise! I didn't expect that, I'm really excited that you feel about me this way, I wouldn't mind it, if it wasn't for the distance. I mean, Germany-Los Angeles!"

Wow, okay, I thought to myself. That actually sounded pretty positive. I told him that I would message him again the next day since friends were coming to visit me. Pure self-protection. Full stop.

"Where did we leave off?" He asked the next day! "Matthews, forget what I said yesterday, it's really a very long distance, how is there supposed to be any future for us?" I replied.

"No, don't say that, if you say that and then take it back ... it's been said and I think it's wonderful! You said it and it touches me, so either you're coming to Los Angeles or I'm coming to Germany for Christmas and New Year's Eve and see you there!"

"I'm coming to Los Angeles this summer!" I said firmly. This time I wouldn't miss any opportunity.

I already dreamed of Matthews, how we would walk down the beach together. Hand in hand on the long beaches of Santa Monica, all the way to Malibu ...

I imagined the beautiful scenery of the pier of Santa Monica with the ocean, street performers and the most beautiful sunsets I have ever seen in my life. Sealed with a kiss. Several kisses ...

"Wow, okay, I'm really looking forward to it, when you visit, I'll show you some of the most beautiful restaurants in Los Angeles and we'll listen to jazz music at home, with a nice bottle of wine. Then we'll catch up with what we missed in Paris." I wonder what he meant with that?

...He continued, "But you have to know one thing. I'm sharing my big apartment at the Walk of fame with a woman; with a roommate!"

What? I thought, a woman? What was that supposed to mean? How should that ever work out? And why did he share his apartment?

"What, with a woman?" I asked directly!

"LOL," he replied ... "She's hardly home.

We know each other here from LA. She is not my type at all and always traveling! Don't worry about it!"

Okay, so I calmed down and didn't think about it any further ...

If only someone had told me then that this was going to be the biggest mistake of my life so far!

Los Angeles

"Dear passengers, this is the flight to Los Angeles, I am your captain and I wish you a good flight."

Okay, now it was actually happening. I was on my flight to Matthews to LA. My excitement was still limited, but that would change soon if I just got to be close to him. I have been to Los Angeles before. It was extraordinary. The first time, I already fell in love with the city and the people there!

Compared to Germany, there's a huge difference in LA: America, the whole lifestyle of the people in fact, is generally different!

The friendliness and openness of the people in America even reminded me of the humor and open-mindedness of the people from Russia! I am Russian myself, born in Siberia and I could never really call Germany my home.

Unfortunately, I have always lacked the warmth and openness of the people I have been looking for in vain in the country. In Russia, there were big festivals and big gestures among the people and neighbors - which is becoming increasingly rare in Germany.

Sadly, people are always fixated on the bad things and what they could do even better than others. In America, I felt a different energy that was already catching up at the airport, along with the better weather! Most times around the year, the sun was shining, maybe that's why people were more enthusiastic and had a happier and more open mindset. The big difference between America and Germany is that you can present what you have achieved in America! You don't have to hide it. In Germany, unfortunately, there are always a lot of people envying your success! You can also make friends really fast in America. Sometimes these friendships are brief, other times, they last for a life time! But as you know, everything has two sides to the medal in life ...

I was watching a block buster, it actually was a really long flight. There was a very nice woman sitting next to me. She traveled with her mother. The woman was around 60 years old. We talked for a while. She started telling me about her life and that she would visit her son in Los Angeles. I told her about Matthews and Bill.

Yes, Bill was the director. We messaged each other for a few days before my flight, he told me he wanted to meet up with me for a coffee. Meanwhile, Bill had met a woman and was firmly in love with her, which made me really happy for him.

I showed her the picture of Matthews. "That's a handsome young man!" Yes, he was. We drank wine together to combat my nervousness.

The captain's voice was suddenly reaching us through the microphone, "In less than 30 minutes, we'll land in Los Angeles!" Oh my god, I couldn't even begin to put in words how excited I was ...

Matthews would pick me up from the airport with his car! I really hoped that both of our expectations would be met. After we landed and I grabbed my baggage, I quickly walked to the exit of the airport. I was so excited about Matthews. How would it be between us in Los Angeles? Was the spark the same as in Germany and Paris? Actually, I knew next to nothing about this man! But now it was too late for any doubts.

I quickly walked towards the exit of the airport L.A LAX. I was so excited. I ran outside and saw a man sitting in a BMW convertible. A white shirt, sunglasses, his black hair fell loose into his face. It was hot in L.A and it was not just the weather!

I took off my jacket. I wore a black top with lace at the neckline underneath. He had a huge grin on his face. It couldn't have been any wider. And I returned the smile! He got out of the car, took my luggage off me and put it in the trunk of his car. "Hi, how do you like the climate here?"

"I love it!" We drove through Los Angeles. There was quite the jam on the highway. We were stuck in traffic for about 2 hours. When we arrived at his house, it was already evening. He parked his car and then we went to his apartment! It was even better than I imagined. It was

120 sqm big with a large garden. Secluded from the outside, not far from the Walk of fame. When you'd leave the apartment, you'd see many big houses and the Hollywood Sign in the distance.

I felt an indescribable energy inside of me! I had never felt like this before in my life. "Would you like to go for a drink at the Hollywood Roosevelt? It's just a few minutes of walking distance away ..."

How could I say no to that, I made myself up after the long flight and we went out. There was nobody at the Walk of fame, since it was the middle of the week and late at night. The famous road lit up in the headlights, a white Lamborghini was parked at the side of the road...

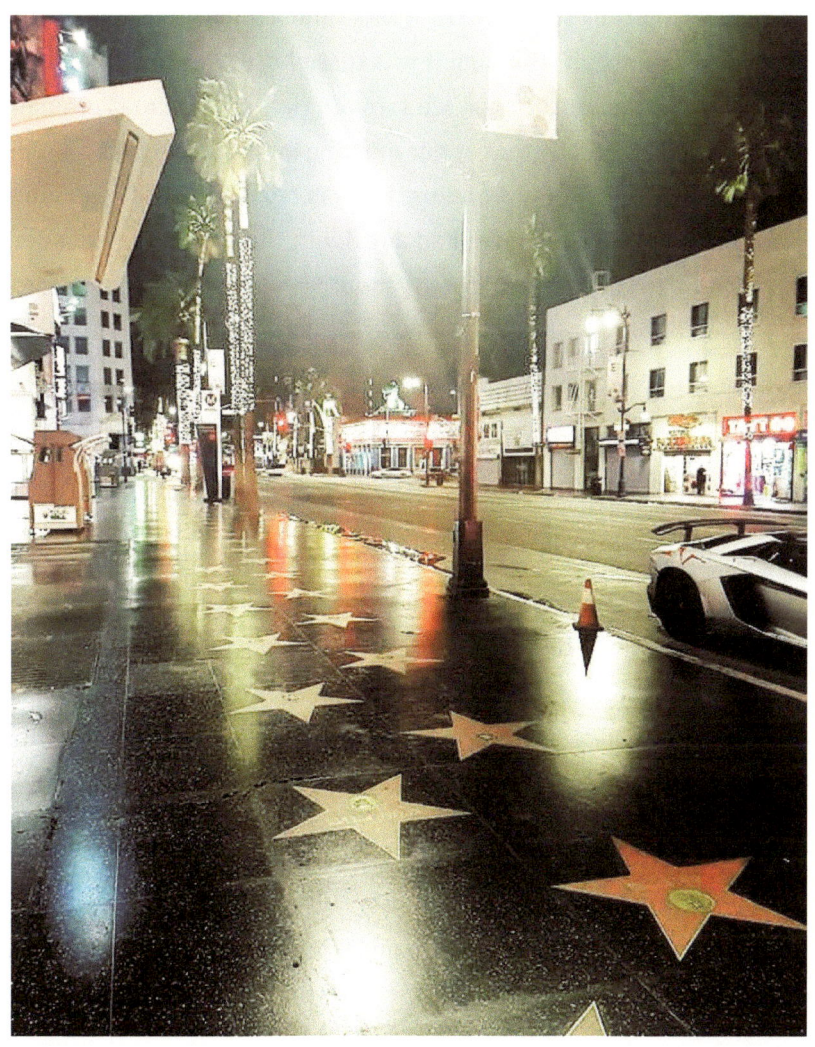

The heat was getting stronger and it was almost unbearable. Eventually, we arrived at the bar. Although it was quite busy, we were able to get two seats. "It was prosecco on ice for you, right?" He actually remembered that. I had exactly that at our meeting in one of the bars we were in. He drank a gin and tonic and the ice was crushed. The conversation took its course and I no longer had any doubt that it was the right decision to come to Los Angeles. I forgot about Richard and Bill, the director. That moment here with Matthews was all that mattered.

We walked back to the apartment past the Walk of fame as he suddenly grabbed me by the arm and pulled me in for a passionate kiss ......

I was in a state of ecstasy as he lied on top of me, moving slowly and gently. I started to moan, he looked deep into my eyes before he kissed me passionately and bit my lower lip, then he moved downward to kiss and caress my entire body, I was about to explode ... He roughly grabbed my hair just to gently move his hands through it again short after.

Oh God, I loved this man with every atom of my body. "You are so sexy," a soft voice lovingly whispered into my ear. It was a dream that I never wanted to wake up from. It was my erotic Hollywood dream ...

When I woke up, Matthews was blissfully asleep beside me. I hoped that I hadn't just dreamed that. The night was just incredible. Almost magical, as always, when I was with Matthews.

I got dressed and went to the kitchen to get some coffee.

Suddenly a voice said to me: "Hey I'm Hanna. Nice to meet you!" Oh my God, I had completely forgotten this other woman, how could I? I turned around and looked at Hanna from head to toe. She was prettier than I thought, had light brown curly hair and appeared very friendly yet somehow forced! "Are you enjoying your stay in California?"

"Yes, sure" I replied somewhat insecure and quickly took off. When I got back to the room, Matthews wasn't there anymore. All I found was a note lying on the bed. "I went to the gym, enjoy the day!" Obviously, I had imagined the day after our first night to start differently! I went back to the kitchen, where I met Hanna again.

"I'm going to watch a Thriller Movie at the Cinema. Want to come with me?" "Sure, give me a second!" I disappeared in the bathroom and got myself dressed and ready.

We were busy throughout the morning. We walked past the Walk of fame towards the Chinese Theater to watch the movie. This was followed by a workout in a gym near the apartment. The view was incredible. As we pedaled on the bikes, Hanna told me a lot about the famous Hollywood Sign. Many people had already ended their lives here ...

Hanna was very accommodating towards me, which I found somewhat odd. But maybe that was just how Americans treated strangers. She asked me about my age and was very interested in what type of man I preferred. At the latter, my alarm bells should have been ringing. Maybe they did and I simply ignored them.

Her eyes, the way she looked at me from the side, the way she talked to me- those were the first signs. After a long workout, we went back to the apartment. On the way, I sent Matthews a message that I was out with his roommate. His answer was fleeting, very different from what I was used to. Did something happen? Did I annoy him? Or was Hanna more than just a roommate to him and he kept it a secret from me? If so, was she are that Matthews was having sex with me?

When we came back, Matthews was already waiting for us. The way he greeted Hanna made me feel uncomfortable. So familiar. They whispered, but I couldn't understand what they said.

Matthews seemed generally absent. A thousand thoughts went through my head. Is it over now before it even started properly? Did he play with me, with my feelings? Was I not interesting anymore now that he managed to get me into his bed?

"Hey sorry, I was working out, you know, gotta keep your body fit." He winked meaningfully-"Now I'm all here for you again, what do you want to do, we could cook something, or would you rather go out?"

"Let's go to a nice restaurant," I answered quickly. "I'm just gonna take a quick shower" And then I disappeared into the bathroom. Like everything in America, the bathroom was oversized as well. Jacuzzi, 2 sinks, a shower that simulated summer rain. So far, I've only ever seen something like that in the movies. I felt like I was staying at a 5-star hotel. Pure luxury. I was standing in the shower trying to get Hanna out of my head when I completely unexpectedly felt Matthews hands on my hips. I didn't even notice him entering the bathroom ...

He kissed my neck and my ear ... I turned around and we kissed each other passionately. Him reaching for the remote control seemed so casual, suddenly, jazz music was playing in the background, the light was dimmed.

Oh my God, my whole body was going crazy, it was something I'd never felt before with a man ... I felt like I could touch the lust and the fire that was in the air. He hadn't promised too much.

Things got more and more exciting and wild, he focused on my breasts. I was about to explode, my whole body gave in to him. I fell more and more in love with this man.

How would this story go? He gave me no time to think: He pressed me against the wall and started kissing me wildly and passionately. I would never forget these scenes in the shower. ....

"Now it's probably too late for visiting a restaurant," I said with a grin on my face as we came out of the shower and got dressed.

"It's never to late to visit a good sushi restaurant with a beautiful lady!" He said with a smirk, his perfect English and his throaty voice taking my breath away.

"Let's go, I know the owner of a great sushi restaurant in West Hollywood." This time I chose a red dress with black high heels and bright red lipstick, a jacket wasn't necessary, it was a wonderful, warm night.

We took Matthews convertible to West Hollywood. The restaurant was on a hill. From there, you could see all of Hollywood. It was fantastic. In the middle of the restaurant, there was a large pond, with a huge screen behind it. The owner walked up to us to greet Matthews and me and offered us the best spot right by the pond. It was incredible.

"I think it was really nice with you!" He said. I was almost speechless and I realized how my face started to glow. "I think it was very nice with you, too" I replied. We ordered a large plate of sushi and the best wine.

Of course, everything was free for us, the owner gave Matthews a meaningful smile. Matthews leaned over to me and whispered in my ear "take off your panties." I didn't know what to say, I gave him a piercing look and then I did what he said ...

My entire body was glowing, the chemistry between us was erotic and tense at the same time. After lunch we drove to Downtown Los Angeles. The view was indescribable.

The skylines lit up and all of L.A was shining brightly. It really looked like a city of angels.

"Come with me, I'll show you something!" He took my hand and dragged me along. Into an elevator, all made of glass. His hand moved up under my dress. Just when I started to enjoy the scene, the elevator stopped and we arrived at the top. I couldn't believe my eyes. So many people, all so beautifully dressed. I had to sort my thoughts for a moment as we went outside to the balcony of this roof top bar. From there, you could see Downtown L.A ...

It was all still like a Hollywood movie and I wished it would have gone on forever. I have never been so happy in my life as I was with Matthews and this city was just the cherry on top. It was not just Matthews. The people, the energy, the liveliness that was clearly present. On top of the creativity of the people. All that made Hollywood appear so special.

We ordered a martini and enjoyed the evening. "Emma, I want you to stay longer with me! I really like you, can you do that?"

Wow, I was speechless once again. I didn't know what to answer. Then, without much thought, I said that I really wanted to do that. We held each other's hands and the evening couldn't have gotten any better. Or could it?

When we left the roof top bar, there was still this erotic sense in the air. And Matthews stopped at nothing. While driving, his hand wandered back onto my thigh. Slowly he moved his hand up under my dress, to where my panties should have been. I was breathing heavily and I could barely control myself to not moan out loud in pleasure.

Matthews left the highway and drove the car out of town. "Where are you going?" I wanted to know. "Close your eyes and allow yourself this surprise!" He replied with a wild passion in his voice.

The car stopped, Matthews grabbed my silk scarf and blindfolded me. "Give me your hand, I'll guide you!"

We stopped walking, but Matthews stopped me from taking off the scarf. His hands were everywhere. I felt him brush my dress over my head, burying his face between my breasts as he skillfully opened my bra. I could feel his gentle kisses all over my body as he got more and more wild, more and more passionate. He gently pushed me to the ground, I felt the grass below me as he gently and wildly penetrated me. I moved in a state of ecstasy, my body reared up, demanding more and more until it almost exploded. A dream that I never wanted to wake up from.

I still had no idea what would come soon.

When I woke up, I was lying in Matthew's bed. The place next to me was empty, so I went to the breakfast table first. There was already food on it, everything one could wish for. Matthews, however, was nowhere to be found. Instead, there was a note on the table. "Emma, I'm filming today. Have a nice day. See you later. Last night was incredible! – Matthews"

At the thought of last night, I inevitably turned red and grinned all over my face.

Hanna came out of her room and sat down at the table. I still found it very strange that he shared the huge apartment with a woman. Anyone else would hear alarm bells ringing in this regard. Usually, I would have heard them too, but I was so excited and happy about the situation with Matthews and this city at the same time that I probably just accepted it that way. I was in a frenzy that was never going to end again and my natural alarm system was simply turned off.

"Hi, how are you? Do you enjoy L.A?", Hanna asked cheekily and demanding. But I stayed cool. "Yes, thank you, it's an incredible city!"

"Yes, it is. You should come next time for a longer trip. Well, I have a good camera. We could take some nice pictures at the beach today. Maybe at the Malibu Beach?" I thought the offer was very nice. And a few great pictures of me on the famous Malibu Beach would certainly do well in my collection. "Sounds great!" She suddenly gave me a very friendly smile, and I was relieved about that, after all, it wasn't a bad idea to try and get along with the woman Matthews was living with all year around.

"I still have to do my laundry," she said suddenly and then she was gone. Again, kind of, I thought. I didn't worry about it too much and went to Matthews study room. It was all designed very modern with gray, white metallic colors and yet, the space seemed to radiate the passion that Matthews felt when acting.

I found a script / piece of Romeo & Juliet, also my favorite piece from my past. I saw many parallels between us. Long before I met Matthews, I had a passion for movies, USA and, of course, the city of Los Angeles.

I had visited this city 2 years ago with friends. Before I met Matthews. It was a dream that came true for me. Nevada, Grand Canyon, the vast desert, freedom in the air and a wind that blew into my face. What else did I need to be happy? I have always been fascinated by the creative work of acting. I think it's the only profession where you can take on other roles without having to apologize which was impossible in every-day life situations. When I was 15, I was asked what I wanted to become and I told myself "I want to be an actress".

I had never dared to realize this dream. Meeting someone like Matthews now inspired me to pursue my dream. I saw all the pictures of events on the red carpet, fellow actors and many books about acting as a profession. It inspired and touched me so much that I completely forgot the time. I looked at pictures from the time he studied drama at the prestigious school in New York, New York! New York, this city has always been my dream. A dream that couldn't come true just yet. Maybe soon it could come true with Matthews?

It was already four o'clock in the afternoon when I looked at the clock. Didn't Hanna want to go to the beach to take pictures?

She had suggested to do something - and then preferred to do the laundry all day? I decided to go to the kitchen to check on Hanna and figure this out.

"Let`s go to a store, 5min. away from here, as there is a snack with lots of fresh fruit and frozen yoghurt, the best here!"

She said that as if it was completely normal to just let someone down and then pretend that nothing had happened. I didn't show how weird I found her behavior. "Ok, sounds fantastic, let's go!" I replied slightly irritated.

We went to this place and she really didn't disappoint me regarding the store. It was the best thing I have ever eaten. My mobile phone rang. A message from Matthews. The filming day was over, he would be home soon, I told him that I was with Hanna and we would be back soon, but again, he only responded in a brief matter.

Strange. Whenever Hanna was involved, he was so distant. What was going on with Matthews? I had the feeling that he had a secret and couldn't fully open up to me! Was he really honest with me at any given time? I somehow had a bad feeling. It was just too good to be true. But maybe I just deserved to be happy! And I sure was happy with that moment, with Matthews and with this city!

"Hi, did you have a nice day?" Matthews greeted me when he got into the apartment and kissed me on the lips. "Yes, it was entertaining, how was your shooting day?" I replied.

"It was nerve-wracking. We're not making the kind of progress the producer wants." I noticed a sad undertone in his voice. He bit his lower lip and looked very thoughtful, and I must confess it aroused me!

It was exciting to me how he spoke in perfect English, when he bit his lower lip and looked at me sadly and thoughtfully at the same times! Phew, I had to mentally distract myself before he realized what he did to me. I didn't want to seduce him in this situation. He certainly would have been overwhelmed in this situation. I pushed my thoughts aside and didn't want to see him sad!

"Let's go to the Santa Monica beach, I want to see the sunset with you at the pier!" He gave me a smirky smile, "Let's go, Emma!" I got goose bumps because of his voice every time.

We walked hand in hand along the pier, there were artists everywhere, many tourists, as well as dancing and laughing people. It was just perfect. We walked to the end of the pier, where we sat on a bench to enjoy the sunset. I felt like I was in a dream that should never end.

Next door, close to a café, they played classical music. This evening couldn't have been more beautiful. We didn't talk much, looked each other in the eyes and kissed passionately. My knees trembled and I felt the desire for more.

Suddenly he stopped and seemed as depressed as he just sometimes was! Was it all too much for him? Should I give him some space? I couldn't shake the feeling that something tormented him. "Matthews, is everything okay? You look so depressed today."

"It's fine, it was just a rough day, come on, let's go, I know a good lounge in West Hollywood, we can spend the rest of the evening." He took my hand in a demanding manner and we went to his car. He kissed me again. I returned the kiss passionately. It's crazy what love can do to a person. I had love in mind, but what did Matthews feel for me?

He was very hard to read and understand. Sometimes I felt very close to him and very far away the next moment. Arriving in the lounge, he pulled me towards the dance floor right away.

I could feel how excited he got seeing me dance. We hugged each other and kissed each other passionately and lustfully. Back in the apartment we had sex. Again and again. When I needed to catch my breath, we snuggled up on each other in the jacuzzi, drinking a bottle of champagne. In the background, the song "Linger" by the Cranberries was playing.

I was completely and irrevocably in love with Matthews! I think he knew that. But who could have known that it was going to be our last evening together?

I suddenly woke up in the night. Something had torn me from my dream. A glance at the alarm clock told me it was five in the morning. Far too early to get up.

I looked right over my shoulder. Matthews slept calmly and as deeply as a baby. I didn't want to wake him up. But since I couldn't sleep, I slipped out of bed and went to the open kitchen.

It was a beautiful kitchen island, everything was white. I opened the fridge to see if there was something in there that could satisfy my hunger. I decided for fried eggs.

A noise broke my thoughts. "Hello?" What a cliché response, I thought, but in this moment of horror, there didn't seem to be anything better I could have said. No response. I closed the fridge and slowly walked out of the kitchen when suddenly, Hanna stood in front of me.

"Holy shit!" I yelled out, trying to calm myself. Out of sheer terror, I dropped the eggs which were now spilled on the floor.

What the hell is she doing in the kitchen so early in the morning?

She was still made-up and wore a dress and High Heels. She probably just came home from a long night out. That's what she looked like! I turned on the lights and we cleaned up the disaster together. Matthews didn't need to hear about this incident.

Luckily, he was sound asleep. "I am sorry I came from a party with friends and wanted another snack". Okay, but that didn't explain the weird sneaking around and then her standing right in front of me out of nowhere! Was this intentional? This woman was like a book with seven seals to me ...

She actually looked pretty. Only her nose was too big for a woman's face. But maybe I just didn't want to treat her like she was a pretty woman, because it felt so weird that she was living in an apartment to-gether with Matthews. Of course, I never asked for the background story to that.

She had brown eyes, a slightly darker complexion, slightly wavy coppery brown hair, she was very slim and spoke very fast in English, which is why I understood only half of what she said. I didn't want to appear impolite and get along with her.

According to what she told me, she was from the Dominican Republic, if I understood her correctly. I didn't quite understand what she did for a living. Not even Matthews could tell me. Apparently, it was nothing of importance to her. She mentioned that she wanted to get into Universal Studios to work behind the scenes.

Of course, Matthews said he knew his way in anytime. Obviously, I thought, as an actor in Los Angeles ...

"Where did you meet Matthews?" Hanna asked curiously and interrupted my thoughts. "I met him in Germany" I replied briefly. "Nice!" She said jealously.

I asked her the same ... "I met him here at an event!" she replied. "What kind of men do you like?"

What a question. Why did she want to know that? Didn't she see that I was with Matthews? "I`m looking at the personality. But of course, he should have a certain attractiveness for me."

With that, I wanted to end the conversation. But Hanna talked more and more and about different types of men, which she thought were attractive but stupid or intelligent and less attractive ...

Matthews had both, but was I the only one seeing that? Certainly not. "I`ve lived with a man before but it wasn`t good, I asked him to leave.

With Matthews, it`s really good", she emphasized loudly. I looked at her a little shocked, what was she trying to tell me there?

By now, it was eight o'clock and Matthews joined us in the kitchen. He was dressed sporty and once again, he whispered with Hanna. Unfortunately, when they spoke English with each other, they were too fast and inaudible. I didn't like that.

Again, the weird atmosphere was apparent. Something was wrong here. My gut feeling got worse.

"Emma, I'm gonna do my workout now. Later, I have an appointment with my agent" When he left, I stayed behind without any kiss. I was alone with Hanna again.

"Let`s go to a great club tonight. They play indie house there.

I mean, if you don´t have any plans with Matthews" Hanna said.

I agreed, it seemed reasonable at the time. I felt that Matthews needed his space. I didn't want to give him the impression that I was just fixated on him. "Ok, see you later, bye!" and then she was gone.

I freshened up and walked the 5 minutes to the Walk of fame. It was a hot day. There were artists everywhere, loud music was playing, there were performances and entertainment all over the place. The Walk of fame is a very crazy place.

But sadly, this place wasn't nearly as exciting and beautiful as I've seen it in the Hollywood movies. It was neither clean nor inspiring. There was a scent of something evil and dangerous in the air. Especially if you went to this place in the evening.

I had the feeling that you were supposed to sell your soul to the devil at this place and you did exactly that. It is definitely an impressive place. But also a place full of sadness and shady characters. Hollywood had the whole world under control. Hollywood determined whose dreams and longings are brought to the canvases of this world. This city couldn't be more contradictory. But it also cast a spell on me, I had made a pact with the devil as well ......

The Walk of fame spans 18 blocks on either side of the Hollywood Boulevard. But I only had eyes for the Victoria Secret store and walked right up to it. When I arrived in the apartment hours later, I got ready for the evening. I chose the blue short Chanel dress from my aunt in Paris. The dress she gave me for my birthday when I was with Matthews at the Moulin Rouge. I think that was the night I definitely fell in love with Matthews.

I still had the sound of French music in my head. The music that was played in the restaurant, where we sat in the end, before his departure where we looked deeply into each other's eyes. Lost in thought, I put on my make up with smokey eyes before I put a black jacket over the blue Chanel dress. There was a comfortable couch in Matthew's office, inviting me to relax. There I was lying, thinking about my life, until tiredness overcame me and I closed my eyes.

Matthew's voice woke me up. He was on the phone, apparently with his agent, ignoring me. That voice, I thought. As he spoke English, I couldn't describe it. It still took my breath away.

Then Hanna left the bathroom. In a very short mini skirt, her loose blouse with tiger patterns and the matching high heels, she looked very sexy. "I`m ready, let's go!" She said in a demanding manner.

As I followed her, I tried once again to get a reassuring look from Matthews. But he was still on the phone. However, he gave Hanna's short skirt a sharp look, which suggested that he found her attractive. I didn't like that. What was going on with Matthews? Was there more between him and Hanna? Was I so blind in this story? Was I unlucky in love once again? My gut feeling told me quite loudly not to go out with Hanna ...

But sometimes in life you unfortunately don't listen to your guts like you're supposed to, even if it was already ringing the alarm bells ... My otherwise razor-sharp intuition was clouded by this glamorous glitter and dream world, which I was part of at the moment. It was too late!

"Have fun!" Matthews added briefly! And then we were heading out for the Walk of fame, in fact, we weren't actually walking, we were running, in High Heels. But why we were running, I had no idea, maybe because it was dangerous.

There were a lot of people everywhere. We were approached by every other person until we arrived at the club. We went through the VIP area to meet friends of Hanna. Everything happened very fast. Everything came with free drinks, a cool mood and a breathtaking location. We went to the smoking area, where Hanna exchanged numbers with a famous musician ......

"Do you see how I get to know people here", she added proudly. When we went back to the dance floor, the unbelievable happened, and I started to dance, and all of Hanna's friends flocked around me, women as well as men came up to me and wanted to talk to me and give me compliments!

It seemed like Hanna's friends liked me, a friend of Hanna took me to the higher VIP area of the club, where the DJs were staying too. What an incredible feeling to have a star DJ so close you could touch them. All of this felt like it had so much charm and fulfilling dreams in it.

It was well past midnight when we left the club and went back to the apartment by taxi. When we got out, it happened. Completely without any warning, Hanna screamed at me and told me to leave her apartment.

She just ran away with a hateful look on her face. I ran after her, still in shock and a few feet behind. What did I do to her? And why should I leave HER apartment? I thought that was Matthew's apartment ...

Hanna was already in the house when I finally arrived there out of breath. She opened the door just to slap it in my face.

"I'll tell Matthews everything!" But what did she want to tell Matthews, I hadn't done anything. Did I get along too well with her friends? Did she didn't like that? I was clueless, sad, insecure and frustrated ...

There I stood. In the middle of the night, on the Walk of fame, and just didn't understand what was going on. Everything around me became meaningless. I think that's how several people have felt in this place when they realized that a dream was slowly bursting. A pink balloon from which air and the love slowly escapes.

Should I too suffer this fate ... what was going on here? What kind of game was Hanna playing there? And what role did Matthews play in all of that?

Tears ran down my face and I tried to calm myself down first.

Then I grabbed my mobile phone and called Matthews. Without a word, he opened the door for me and let me in. I didn't feel like talking in that moment. All I wanted was to lay down on the bed in my expensive Chanel dress and sleep. There was no sign of Hanna.

When I woke up the next morning, I had to sort my thoughts out first. My makeup was smeared because of all the tears. I discovered a ring I had received from Hanna's girlfriends. I quickly ran to the bathroom to freshen up and wash the makeup off my face.

"Get out of my apartment, immediately!" I jumped and Hanna stood in the door of her bedroom yelling at me "If it wasn`t for Matthews, I`d have done you a lot more harm!" she threatened with a hateful expression in her face. She raised her hand to slap me but fortunately, I reacted quickly, grabbing her hand in time to stop her. Her expression said it all.

She was very surprised at my strength. She probably underestimated me a bit. "Well," I said calmly, "I think Matthews should also decide, if I have to leave this apartment."

"I will make sure that Matthews will never contact you again!"

With that sentence, she took her bag and walked to the door. "Leave my apartment, today!" And then she was gone, I was so shocked that I didn't know what to say.

Since I didn't know what to do, I went back to the bedroom, to Matthews. He looked at me confused when he saw my tears. "What happened yesterday, Emma?"

"Matthews, I don't know, nothing happened that could justify Hanna's reaction!

I have a question, Matthews. And please be honest with me:

"Is this Hanna's apartment?"

Matthew looked down, he seemed ashamed. He gave me a brief "Yes" and I didn't understand anything at all anymore, was Matthews a complete impostor and liar, or was he just embarrassed to say that the apartment belonged to Hannah, if so, then he could have said so.

There was not the slightest reason to keep that from me. Or was there? Why did he live with her? Was that purely for financial reasons, or did they have a love affair?

No, this couldn't be. That would be impossible ......

"Emma you are an amazing woman and having sex with you ... well, that's just breathtaking. But there can't be any more between us."

He swallowed hard and had tears in his eyes.

I was paralyzed and didn't really buy it.

Then he went on ...

"I have nothing to offer you, Emma. I live here with Hanna, because I could never afford my own apartment in this situation. The roles I've been offered so far aren't that well-paid. And when I start a family, when I get married, then I want to be able to offer something to the woman I love. More than just an apartment I share.

I have goals. I want to become famous internationally. And only then do I want to start a relationship, marry and start a family.

You know, my friend, for example, bought his girlfriend an engagement ring worth $ 50,000. Just because.

If I want to be successful, then the woman on my side should also be an actress! I hope I'm not hurting you now."

Wow, that stung! I am not usually speechless, but now I didn't know what to say. I was so hurt and horrified at the same time. It was a slap in the face that I could hardly handle.

"No, Matthews, it's all ok," I lied. But I couldn't suppress my tears.

He continued...

"If you lived in Los Angeles, we would meet, then we could move together and build a future together, but there is also the distance to it, I
don't want to allow feelings with this distance between us, it just hurts.
This can't work, it just doesn't fit."

I didn't know what to say. Tears streaming down my face, I packed my
bags and waited for the taxi that he had called in the meantime for me.
When I got in, I looked him straight in the eye once again, then the taxi
drove off and only faintly, I saw him vanish from afar. A veil of infinite
grief took over me. Deep inside, I had the feeling that we will never see
each other again ...

In the taxi, the song "Secretly" by Skunk Anansie was playing. Fate didn't
mean well with me. And then I couldn't hold back my tears.

Meanwhile, I booked a flight back to Germany via app and asked the
taxi driver to take me to the airport. I saw no reason to stay here, not
even a day longer.

"What's wrong, honey? I'm Zane. Nice to meet you!"

His gentle voice conjured up a small smile in my face.

"It's a sad love story," I replied.

As if he knew how to cheer me up, he turned on loud hip hop music and turned the car into a private club.

While we drove to the airport, we sang the songs and really had fun. Zane was the most positive person I've ever met. That's exactly what I needed now.

Arrived at the airport, I quickly wiped my tears and powdered my face. Zane helped me with the suitcases and gave me something small.

"Bring it back to me when you come back to Los Angeles!" When I looked at my hand, there was a USB stick with a love song collection, I hugged him and said, "Sure, thank you!" Before I left, we quickly exchanged numbers and then I went to the terminal quickly, my flight took off in 45 minutes and the boarding had already begun.

I was grateful that I could get a window seat. I had the opportunity to look out the window. The last few days passed by in my thoughts again. Sad as I was, I looked at my phone and there was actually a message from Matthews.

As I listened to the song "Colorblind," I read the message he had sent. "I wish you a good flight. I am very sorry that I didn't get to bring you to the airport. I had to film and our producer tolerates no delay at the moment. Although it was a strange constellation, I really enjoyed our encounter. Greetings, Matthews."

Ok, I thought. A "strange constellation". I didn't know what to answer and looked out the window. When the next song "Ordinary Life" by the Weekend was played on my headphones,

I turned off my phone with a tear on my face. Although I was completely upset inside, I fell asleep immediately and only woke up when we reached Germany already.

When I opened my eyes, people on the plane were already in the corridors, waiting to be let out.

I had a bad dream, I had lost the man I loved. Oh no, that was reality. I sorted out my thoughts briefly and joined the waiting queue.

While I hurried to get to the baggage handling, everything was just blurry around me. I ignored the crowd, I was caught in a parallel world. A world of pain and sorrow. The love of my life had disappeared from my it ....

Berlin

I had just closed my apartment door behind me when my mobile phone notified me of an incoming message. It was Matthews. "Emma, I hope you have arrived well. I'm worried about you. I could hardly focus at the set. Things got weird, let's have a talk tomorrow.

I .... "

It was a very long text. And since it was now 4 o'clock in the morning, I had no desire to read the entire message. I was dead tired but couldn't sleep. I wasn't sure what I should answer him or whether I should answer at all. Maybe I should forget about him and be done with it. This love for him would otherwise destroy me inside.

But since I couldn't accept how I felt just yet, I decided to answer with a short message at least.

"Matthews, I'll get in touch. OK? Emma" And as soon as I sent the message, his picture disappeared, he just completely deleted me!

I couldn't hold back my tears, the pain, the anger, and started crying aloud. With a force, I slammed my phone against the wall. It broke, just like my entire life was broken.

But the pain remained deep inside of me. My life had turned into a movie. A film without action and without a leading actress. I wasn't part of it anymore. Everything around me was just moving on automatically, without me.

The summer was coming to an end. Autumn came, then it was winter. The months passed by and I tried to get back to my everyday life here in Germany. I was no longer myself. I felt like a robot. There was no sign of life coming from Matthews.

He disappeared and so did I along with him.

The months went by, and almost unnoticed, spring was just around the corner. And Matthews? I just couldn't forget about him. To distract myself, I decided to visit Vanessa in Zurich. We talked a lot. I told her about Matthews, about my time in L.A.

And about Hanna and being kicked out of the apartment. "Sweetie" she said affectionately, "maybe there was in fact something going on between them and she just allowed him his freedom. Who knows what all this was about. Eventually, you would have moved to L.A. and what would have happened then? Imagine this would have happened when you already had moved there. In a completely foreign city, without any support."

"You're right!" I admitted thoughtfully. "Slowly but surely, I have to let go. This is in the past now. I have to get my life back on track again!"

So, I decided to participate in a make-up artist and acting workshop in Berlin!

Since I had relatives in Berlin, I could probably stay at their place. I would be able to live with my relatives during the workshop.

And in order to make progress in my career, I had to do something anyway. So, I signed up for the workshop and finally, I had a goal that was worth working towards to again.

The course took place in May and was a set-up workshop for editorial shootings for experienced make-up artists.

And as fate would have it, I met Ava there, a well-known make-up artist who had already worked with many celebrities. She told me a short time later that she has an office in the middle of the Hollywood Walk of Fame and that she would commute between LA and Berlin.

Oh man, there was the Walk of Fame again. Did I never get rid of the memories of Matthews? Would he persecute me all my life?

I tried to ignore my memories to suppress the painful world of thought and focused on the conversation with Ava. We got along very well from the start and had the idea to fly to Los Angeles soon. A couple Ava was friends with had a clubhouse on Venice Beach where us four could spend time together. Apparently, all roads led to Los Angeles - no matter where I went.

At the workshop, I was assigned a beautiful model for the photo shoot. I was allowed to make her up in a drama and editorial look, which I enjoyed a lot. We received lots of advice and the workshop was more than successful. I learned a lot and was finally back from the dead. That definitely gave me a motivation boost.

The meeting with Ava gave me the new hope that I needed in order to look optimistically towards the future.

We kept close contact and met regularly. Work connected us and so we always had something to talk about.

Ava let me join for her jobs frequently and introduced me to the Berlin High Society. It was an incredible feeling.

And then there was also the acting course I signed up for...

The dream to become an actress started early in my life and became a vision in L.A., but I was also able to follow my dream here in Berlin.

I was already 30 minutes late when I finally arrived at the film acting school. It was dark inside. Quietly, a light stomping penetrated the silence. The woman on stage performed a well-rehearsed and quite emotional piece and received a good amount of applause from the approximately 10 spectators.

"Hello, please introduce yourself to us!" the lecturer said and nodded to me. "Uh, yes, so first of all, sorry for being late, I sort of underestimated the traffic here and well, once you get into the rush hour...

Well, my name is Emma, I'm a make-up artist, dancer and choreographer. But first and foremost, I work as a make-up artist. I have my own beauty salon with 3 employees. The desire to start acting has grown in me while I was in L.A. I visited an actor there who lives directly at the Walk of fame and I was allowed to get a bit of an insight into Hollywood.

It was incredible. And well, now I would like to learn this wonderful skill and slip into other roles myself."

Only after I had said all this, I realized what I had actually achieved so far. I had built my own existence out of nothing. With diligence, discipline, positive thinking and a lot of stamina. And that wasn't always easy on me.

"Great, I'm looking forward to seeing your performance tomorrow!" the lecturer said. He himself was an experienced actor who wanted to pass on his skills to young talents and was therefore active as a lecturer. Somehow, he was also a bit of a funky guy. He didn't look particularly attractive, rather boring in fact. His toenails were painted in different colors. Each nail in a different color to be exact. Was that supposed to reflect his creativity? He handed out our monologues to us and the first evening was over.

I went back to my relatives. The dinner was ready when I arrived. "You're right on time, Emma. Sit down with us. We were just about to eat." My aunt smiled at me and poured me a glass of wine.

"You should move to Berlin. You'd have great potential here. You could be really successful" the husband of my grand cousin said. "I agree with him, you could look for an apartment in Berlin and until you find something you can live with us." my aunt agreed.

"Thank you, that's so sweet of you. I will think about it and if necessary, get back to this amazing offer. I' quite tired at the moment. See you guys tomorrow morning."

I got up from the table and went to my room. Here, I was finally able to relax a bit and prepare my monologue. But the memories of Matthews were awakened again. And as if he had guessed, my mobile phone rang just in that moment.

"Hello Emma, how are you? Matthews"

The mere thought of him spread goosebumps all over my body. He got back in contact with me. But at what cost should I get involved with him now?

I put away my documents and thought about the time we spent together. The nights with him. The hours of conversation as we walked along the Santa Monica Pier. There it was again, the longing that plagued me and tore me apart inside.

Just when I wanted to answer him, my phone rang. Matthews called. I was shocked and irritated at the same time! What should I do? I only just started to feel better.

Why would you tear up old wounds again, I thought to myself! I waited for the ringing to stop and answered the SMS instead. I let him know that I was fine and that I was working on my monologue I had to study for acting school. I attached a picture of my documents to the message.

„Awesome!" He replied, "I miss you, Emma!"

How was I supposed to answer that? He had hurt me so much. After our last encounter, my life was a sheer mess and it took me many months to regain my balance and clear the rubble left from the suffering and disappointment. While I was thinking about what I should answer and whether I should even answer him at all, I fell asleep. With my documents in hand. It was all too much for me.

When I woke up, I still had my clothes on. My phone blinked. Again a message from Matthews. What I read took my breath away - again:

"I do not know who you are or what you want. I saw your number in Matthews Cellphone. I am his girlfriend, I date Matthews since last summer. So please leave him alone. I don´t want you to contact him anymore. Never again I want to see a message from you!"

That was clear; I didn't understand anything at all anymore. I put away my monologue and started to cry. I cried all night, unable to focus on the monologue; I couldn't even fall back asleep anymore. Not a minute.

Who the hell was that? Maybe Hanna, who would just wanted to step in again and tear us apart forever?

Was there another woman now? And why did this woman, whoever she was, see me as competition? I had not had any contact with Matthews for almost a year. What kind of sick game was this?

First, he told me how much he missed me and then there's a message from "his girlfriend"? I just couldn't suppress my sadness. I was completely down. Again, everything was mixed up.

All this burdened me so much, and now, of all times, when my own life was about to start again. Myself and my life have been pushed into the background by others – and I never asked for it. How did I deserve all of that?

Again, I was too late. Again, I had to hurry so much that I was completely out of breath when I entered the drama school hall. The first participant of the course was currently presenting her monologue. She screamed and cried. Her emotions seemed so real. She was good. Luckily this wasn't a competition. Otherwise, I would have turned back right there and run away. Above all, she knew the script!

"So Emma, it's your turn now! I'm really looking forward to seeing your performance!", The lecturer sneered.

"I'm sorry, I don't fully memorize my script, is it okay if I read it?"

"Yes, that's not a problem, you can also recite it to the point you can memorize it." I swallowed slowly and then the stage fright came in. The lecturer, and also the students, looked at me intently.

"That has always been my dream, I always wanted to die together with my sweetheart, at the same time. So, I could only imagine dying with all of you together. That one of us would leave before the other did, I never would have ...." I stopped and looked at the script ...

I couldn't remember the text, was completely unfocused and bitter. Matthews was omnipresent in my thoughts once again. That got me off track. The thought of last night's news drove me crazy ...

"No problem, Emma. Start again from the beginning!"

This time I read the text. That seemed safer to me. My thoughts would just keep wandering off again and again.

"Thank you Emma!" the lecturer said. I sat down discontented and sank into my dream world. The text I chose was about a woman saying good-bye to her parents with a final video. In the video, she announced that she was no longer interested in life.

She, too, had had everything. She had an affair with a Hollywood star, had traveled the world. She had experienced everything she had ever dreamed of. But she just didn't want to live anymore. A very emotional piece, I think. It reflects a part of my own life.

When everyone was done, I once again went to the lecturer to talk to him! ...

"I would like to ask how I can get started in acting?" Maybe the question wasn't detailed enough. But he just rolled with it and replied:

"Emma, it's a tough business, I'm telling you that. I've never been to Hollywood before, but I've already had some gigs, acting is tough and most of the actors are shuffling from gig to gig and they keep worrying about financials. There's only a small percentage of all actors actually becoming really famous who have chosen this path for themselves at some point. Take me as an example I already had some really good roles. But eventually, things went down. At the moment, I'm in a rather bad spot when it comes to gigs.

That's why I focus more on teaching. I'm just too bad for Hollywood. Emma, it's more likely to win a lottery than to make it to Hollywood. I can tell you that much.

Do that, what's the name, make-up artist thing. You're probably more successful with that."

Well, that's just great This day couldn't get any worse, I thought to myself. What did I expect? My first starring role in a Hollywood blockbuster? But what the lecturer said was very contradictory in my opinion.

That he himself as an actor was unsuccessful was sort of obvious. But what was he trying to tell his students? It seemed to me as if he only did the lecturer's job half-heartedly.

And then, the next tragedy came in. All participants of the workshop were accepted for the first semester for next year at the most renowned drama school in Hamburg. All except me.

I didn't understand the world anymore. I didn't actually score that bad. After all, as a choreographer, I had a really good body feeling. Unlike most others. Wasn't that necessary for an actor? Depressed, I sat in the subway and drove back to my aunt ...

And as if the day didn't come with enough bad news, my aunt announced another shock.

The husband of my grand-cousin had died this morning. Without any warning. There wasn't any information on what had happened. It could happen so fast, next moment, life was over. It was an incredible shock. How much suffering did I have to endure?

How could I survive this? Where should I take my strength from?

I stayed until the funeral, then left Berlin for the time being to concentrate on my work as a make-up artist and choreographer. But I felt this emptiness inside of me. The emptiness I felt after losing the love of my life. A void that nothing and nobody could fill.

Nobody, except Matthews. But why did all my relationships fail until then? What was the reason for this? To identify the cause, I had to go back many years in time. Back to my roots ...

Who am I?

I am Emma. I was born in Siberia / Novosibirsk in Russia. As far as I can remember, I had a happy and carefree childhood.

My memory appears to be really good, since I was only 5 years old when we had to move away from there. My parents both worked full-time and so, my older sister mostly looked after me. My father was an engineer and the passionate lead singer of a band. When I was a small child, he spent 6 months on a ship in the Antarctic. I remember his stories well. In my memories, I imagined the polar sea in the most beautiful variants and colors. My dad could describe everything so figuratively, I almost felt like I had been there myself.

I can still remember my time in kindergarten. I was a very popular child, even had an admirer. When it was time to say goodbye, many tears were shed. I didn't want to leave, I wanted to stay with my friends, in my home country.

But my parents had made this decision. The preparations were made, everything was ready.

The next day, early in the morning, the long journey to Germany began.

I wasn't happy about moving to Germany. The very thought of having to live in another, foreign country made me extremely sad. I had the feeling that I was torn from my roots and suffered quite the trauma as a child.

Actually, I have always been a very happy and clever child that was always up for anything fun.

The years went by, but it didn't get better. "With time, you will get used to your new environment!" My dad told me. "Everything will be better in Germany."

Unfortunately, he was wrong. My mother couldn't handle moving and being forced to leave her homeland, she suffered from severe depression. This serious illness, which could make a person almost feel incapacitated, had sneaked into our family several generations ago. My grandmother and my great-grandmother already dealt with it.

And I too, now a teenager, felt the first symptoms creeping up on me. I, who once was so cheerful, who had loved to learn and was extremely ambitious, lost the desire to live.

I couldn't get myself to study anymore, I wasn't interested in those many fake friendships. My relationship with my sister became more and more difficult, as well.

What happened? I decided that Germany probably didn't suit our family and blamed the move to Germany for all these difficult years we had.

My grandfather, whom I loved more than anything else, died from lung cancer a few years later and my grandmother died from her depression three years later. She was so sick that one day she just stopped eating. Nobody could convince her that she had to eat to stay alive. Nobody could help her, not even the doctors. Her marriage with my grandfather wasn't always easy for her, but she didn't do well with his death.

Their marriage got worse and worse with the years since we lived in Germany. They quarreled almost every day when I visited which was really sad to see, especially if you can't do anything about it. Where was the harmony?

Even the families of my parents didn't get along at all.

What happened in Russia? Why was there so much hatred between the two families? Where was I in this whole family mess? I myself was always looking for some specific type of support and love in order to start my own family. I was convinced that real love had to be out there somewhere. But the only thing life gave me up to this point, was superficial and pointless encounters that didn't emotionally give me what I was looking for so desperately.

It is often said that you have to love yourself first in order to be loved by others! But where do you get this feeling from, if you didn't get it at home? How are you supposed to develop feelings for something you never knew to begin with?

What helped me was working on myself. It involves a lot of discipline, empathy and a great deal of insanity.

Our life has increasingly become a major disaster. Instead of better, as my father repeatedly emphasized after our move, things got worse and worse. The years of dissatisfaction and disharmony took their course. There were constant arguments taking place at the dining table and everyone wanted to prove to the other that they were the better. Everyone wanted to be right, no one was right about anything. Everyone was just trying to win, even if that meant you had to backstab each other.

I had always tried to stay out of the quarrels as best I could. Often, I was nothing but a silent participant in this family tragedy. I didn't know what could have helped. I couldn't do anything to improve the situation. And that's why I simply didn't say anything.

Even at school, it was quiet around me. Unfortunately, I didn't think the school system worked well. I felt like they taught us too little about the things that were needed later in life. Neither the potential of the individual nor the intelligence of the children were promoted.

There were, in fact, people in my life who looked at me like an uncut rough diamond. Unfortunately, these people were very rare in my environment.

If you are constantly surrounded by people who know nothing better than to start arguing and humiliating each other, you will eventually feel inferior yourself.

And so, the self-doubt in me spread more and more.

I managed talk less and less to my father. Constantly, there were misunderstandings, we constantly talked past each other. Living with him became more and more difficult and complicated.

And then I discovered my passion for dance and art.

With a school friend, I studied a choreography, which was later performed with a whole group on stage in our auditorium in front of the whole school. We received so much applause that it inspired us and encouraged us to continue.

Besides the sport, the dancing, I loved to express my feelings with drawing. Almost everything my thoughts dealt with, I put down on paper.

I was already a very creative person back then. Later, this passion should be my vocation and open the door to a better life for me. But until then I had a long, arduous journey ahead of me.

When my parents finally had a solid financial base, we moved to a big house. We had the hope that our family life would calm down if we had more space and weren't stuck with each other so closely anymore. But that was just wishful thinking. This move didn't turn around the constant quarrels either.

I couldn't handle all of this anymore. Why was my life so difficult? Why could I just not find to myself?

At just 17, I slipped into a bad depression. I started drinking, going to parties and having encounters with the wrong men; those who didn't do me any good. Even my so-called "friends" were not what I needed. I searched for the meaning of life and slowly lost myself more and more in alcohol and senseless parties. How would my story continue? Was my fate to die of depression at the age of 30?

No, I said to myself! I certainly didn't want to end up like that. It was time that someone finally tore this chain and didn't allow our family to die of depression.

I grabbed the newspaper and looked for ways to boost my creativity. If no one else did, then I had to take that into my own hands. And there it was. The ad I had searched for so long. A beauty school advertised vacancies.

That was just right for me. A state-approved beautician. Writing the application was a breeze. And when I finally received the letter of confirmation, I was so incredibly happy I could have cried.

One of our first tasks was to pick a book and present it during the next lesson.Not an easy task for me. The only book I ever read was Romeo & Juliet. But that was not exactly what I wanted to introduce.

I motivated myself and made my way to the nearest bookstore. And there it was! The book immediately caught my eye.

"Imagine how it works! He who thinks positively is happier life!"

What a title. I bought the book and headed home. Since I had to drive a bit, I used the time on the bus to start reading. I was so absorbed that I almost missed my exit.

The book captivated me. Reading, I ran home from the bus stop, sat down in my room and read on until I finished the book. And I already felt that day that this book would change my life.

I had one goal in mind. I wanted to become a make-up artist. And the book helped me with that. Slowly, I managed to fight my way out of the depression. I completed the training as a make-up artist without any issues and from then on, there seemed to be only one way to go: the way up!

I fell in love with an attractive man, made many new friends and became very successful with my very own beauty salon.

My secret? A simple formula from the book: visualize your goals!

Regardless of how ambitious your goals are, regardless of what you have to do to achieve them. Keep your goals in mind and you will reach them. I had reached my goal. But that also showed me in what environment I lived.

I was surrounded by jealousy. Jealousy within the family that didn't cope with my sudden success. Jealousy among friends who didn't think I deserved my success. Hate, obstacles and manipulation kept getting in my way. And in the middle of it all, there was always my sister. A driving force that tried to destroy everything that was important to me.

I couldn't understand why. Why was I back at the same point I was at years ago? Did the book only help to a certain extent? Was that it? Was our destiny predetermined from birth? No! I was convinced that wasn't true. I have always believed that we determine our own fate. But without a certain teacher or a good companion, the whole thing turns out to be quite difficult.

Already as a child I had a lot of empathy and a sensational knowledge of human nature. My intuition was very strong and I often felt like things were going to happen that actually did happen then. Unfortunately, with my environment, I was among people whose lives were marked by pragmatics and rejection. This made me become a very lonely person. Even when I was surrounded by a lot of people. You can be in a room full of people and still feel incredibly lonely.

You might even feel this lonely if you are in a relationship with the wrong person.

I think that's just the challenge of our time. A time that is very fast-paced and where very many relationships fail very quickly. People don't take time to catch their breath. Or they get rid of others based on outer features, rather than paying attention to the inner values of a person.

The biggest challenge is to be alone. But this very solitude is often necessary to find oneself. Find out who you really are. Where you come from and where you want to go. Everyone always says you should listen to your guts, which is perfectly right! But how is that supposed to work if you are constantly suppressed by external bad influences!

It's very important to distance yourself from anything bad that stops you from being successful in your life. Even if that means you are lonely at first.

You should have the strength and the will to never doubt your own dreams. Even when others do it all the time and society want to keep you small all the time so you don't grow and become independent! Because independence means strength and success.

When I read the book "Imagine how it works! He who thinks positively is happier life!", my life changed bit by bit for the better. I started to see things positively. I visualized my goals as if they had already arrived and felt an unwavering faith in myself!

I believed in myself and my goals. That I was going to reach them. How things would be if I had already reached my goals. At that time, I met my former partner Mike. A great man, but no idea what it meant to visualize things. My sister started talking to me about how Mike was not the right person for me. She started to talk badly about the relationship. But why did she do that?

Gosh, why did I allow myself to be so negatively influenced by just any-one? Presumably, because I've had no support all my life and even had to play the psychologist for my mother instead of just being a child. I also felt that the negative things dominated our whole family and pulled me down like an anchor.

But I didn't let go of my relationship with Mike and eventually moved in with him.

We treated ourselves to the most beautiful holiday trips and traveled the whole world. But even then, I could feel an increasingly dominant dissatisfaction growing inside of me!

My sister's words kept ringing in my ears. Words that didn't let me go. What if she was right? Or did she use spiritual arson? Was it her inten-tion to disrupt my life?

She was completely in control of me, but I didn't realize that at the time. Apparently, my misfortune mostly started with her. She dominated my subconscious. Because as soon as I thought about her words, the mis-fortune happened.

After much deliberation, I decided to start my own business. Mike wasn't very enthusiastic about this step and tried to talk me out of it. My parents also had their objections and talked to me.

My sister was against everything I did, arguing that these two things didn't go together, career and a relationship. That couldn't work. She staunchly supported this opinion. But on the other hand, she would support me with the idea of opening my own beauty salon. I was indecisive and pretty much alone with everything. Mike and I increasingly distanced ourselves from each other.

It was always the same story. Nothing lasted for eternity except my sister's poison that she purposely or unintentionally spread in my life.

Despite all the resistance and being convinced by my idea to work independently, I began the search for the appropriate premises. I set up my business plan to get grants for my beauty salon. Mike was mostly at the PC during this time. Throughout the night he played his video games.

But I didn't let that stop me. I fought on and it seemed like the fight was worth it. The business plan served its purpose and I received the confirmation for the much needed grants. I just couldn't find the right premises. It was like a curse. And then, after a long, almost endless search, I finally found premises that seemed to be perfect. Immediately after the visit, I got a verbal confirmation from the landlord. But only to get a cancellation a week later. That's the way life goes sometimes.

And again, I was there where I never wanted to be again. Where my life has been so often. In the abyss. It pulled the ground off below my feet and I felt like I was falling into an infinitely deep hole. At that moment, I didn't want to live anymore.

It couldn't go on like that. And apparently it wasn't going to. Plunged in my mind, I drove down the street. I didn't have the slightest desire to go to my sister's birthday. But I couldn't do that to her. Or rather, I couldn't do it to myself. She would remind me of this for years if I didn't appear at her party on a day so important to her.

... Suddenly a bang, my car flipped, I didn't know what side was up. I rolled over and slammed my car against the guardrail.

When I was able to regain my consciousness, firefighters were just getting me out of the car with a cutting device. I couldn't move my legs that were stuck and I was completely paralyzed.

As if from afar, I kept crying out. The people around me were hectic, fire department, police, the ambulance. Everyone was there to rescue me from the car and take care of me. When I finally got out of the car, I saw the whole disaster. Obviously, I collided with a truck. My car was completely crashed. The fact I made it out alive was a miracle.

And that I got away with just a whiplash injury was even more of a miracle. The fact that this terrible accident happened the day of my sister's birthday was very mysterious and incomprehensible at the same time. However, I had a very good protector ...

If anyone else had been driving behind me, this definitely would have been the death of me. As grim as this whole situation was, it was so valuable for my future life.

One could have thought that I was somehow capable of conjuring evil just with my thoughts. And that's what reminded me of the book. Think and attract the positive!

I overcame my depressive episode and did everything I could to recover quickly from my accident. The time I spent lying on the sofa or in my bed I used to read more books, The Secret and Murphy, and to re-motivate myself.

But something was preventing me from moving forward at that moment. Almost as if an unseen force wanted to hold me down with all its strength. Mike! Slowly but surely, it dawned on me why I couldn't make the leap to the top.

Mike was always making me feel bad for anything that happened.

After the accident he complained that I can't drive properly and that the accident was my fault. In general, I was too stupid and incapable of anything. I would too rarely took, not look as attractive as I did in the beginning and I should please leave him alone with the fixed idea to become self-employed, that wasn't going to work out anyway. But when he slapped me in the middle of a fight in a way that I had a head-ache the next day, I just moved out without further ado. It was enough forever!

That meant I had to go back to my parents, at least temporarily, but I gladly took that.

But even if I seemed satisfied with myself externally, I was inwardly so agitated like I hadn't been in ages. When I arrived at my parents, I closed my room's door, leaned against it from the inside and dropped to the floor. What a failure! I was completely devastated and had to regain my strength.

Also, when I actually knew how my parents thought about the plans to open up my own beauty salon, I sat in the living room with them that evening and talked about this topic, hoping to get them to change their minds and get them to my side.

But what they said only dragged me down further. They strongly advised against it. I wasn't going to make it, that it was too much work and I should rather pay attention to my health.

But maybe I would come to my senses if I tried it first. They provided me with their largest basement room and I was able to start attracting customers there for the time being. With the money I had from the promotion, I gradually got the necessary furniture. Since I wanted to work full-time, there was a lot I needed.

And then, that's what I had been dreaming of all the time. I was found by interested parties. And as my clients were so happy with my work, my customer base grew by referral marketing alone. The money flowed and so I was able to work my way up.

Soon after, I finally found suitable premises. With a landlord who believed in me and my success.

The new studio was a dream. Large windows allowed for a lot of sunlight. The three rooms were ideal for spatially separating the various offers. I offered the complete all-round feel-good package. The satisfaction of my customers made word and I soon had a considerable customer base.

Yes, it was hard work, but it paid off. I loved my customers and the customers loved me. It was a give and take. And soon I was so busy that I could hire my first employee.

I didn't regret the step into self-employment until today. That was the best decision I had ever made in my life.

Meanwhile I have three employees. Since my dad knows the bookkeeping stuff quite well, he is managing the premise and I can focus on the essentials.

That's the way it happens sometimes. At first no one believes in you - later you work together side by side. You just have to trust yourself and constantly go your own way.

I always made sure that I was well educated and attended courses and seminars to be always up to date.

The training as a make-up artist completed my education. I was really proud of myself.

And then I finally made it. One day, I got a job that put my professional life to the next level and the last step was initiated:

A well-known, large radio station hosted a fashion show. And they actually asked me if I had the capacity to attend the event and do the make-up of the models. Wow!

What a recognition and a great honor, finally, my professional life was perfect. There was only love left, which was yet to come. But then Richard came ...

Richard

Richard, what a man. Big muscular build, educated and in love with me head over heels. But I didn't make it easy for him in the beginning, he had to fight with all means necessary to get me. And he did that with devotion. After all that I had gone through with Mike, Richard seemed to be the most loving and strongest person I had ever met.

But the relationship between me and my sister became more and more difficult and overshadowed my new relationship. She was a very creative person and was good at dancing and singing. She took part in many beauty contests and also won some of them. We always got along well as long as something went badly in my life.

But as soon as things got better, she was the most venomous, toxic snake. She railed against each of my friends, against my partners, chafing and chopping away at everything I did in life.

I loved my sister more than anything, but these taunts and intrigues made it extremely difficult for me to enjoy my life. Unfortunately, when my life started to get better, she started disrupting it again.

Sometimes I had the feeling she was building me up just to knock me back down right after. Life with her was a constant competition that she always tried to win!

I was not interested in winning. I just wanted to live. To express my creativity, to be able to show my personality openly. I wanted harmony and I wanted success for her, I thought she had talent and we were supposed to support each other.

But whenever I returned to the good side of things in life, she interfered with her hostility. She didn't seem to realize how much this hurt me. What did she want to do with it? What was she trying to do there? Was she trying to make sure I would always be one step behind her? Always in her shadow?

Above all, she was so deceitful. That made it even harder because she played the loving sister on the outside and always complimented me. But what she did, what she did to me, her taunts, her hostilities, said something else.

When I got engaged to Richard, it was almost the end of the world for her. She was so angry that she couldn't even congratulate me on my engagement.

She couldn't handle the idea of me making friends, my choreography, according to her, was the worst she had ever seen. She always drew all the attention to herself, away from me. She tried to keep me in her shadow. No matter what we were doing.

Why was she so hostile? I don't know. To this day, I can't tell what made her be like this.

I was so hurt by her actions that I distanced myself more and more from her. I built up walls that nobody could manage to tear down. I couldn't talk about it to anyone and so the years went by without these walls being removed.

As much as I tried, relationships and friendships only occured just to break down on these walls I had built around me.

My actually happy nature was more and more overshadowed by depression.

Slowly, I started realizing that my depression was not just about our move to Germany. It wasn't purely genetic. Surely the tendency to develop a depression was inherited, so that it could break out, but it was related to something quite different.

My sister had certainly done her part.

But who was capable of tearing down these high walls? Did I have to do it myself before a man could find a place in my life? How could I forget all the pain and all the suffering I had experienced and just move on?

When Richard asked me to become his wife, I was the happiest woman in the world. I loved him and he loved me.

We got engaged after only 3 months relationship. He gave me a huge diamond, which now adorned my left ring finger. Our faces beamed. I finally found my luck.

I was sure: it was him! My soulmate. It was love at first sight! Immediately after the engagement, we decided to move together. He often took me to Spain. There he had a wonderfully beautiful finca by the sea. What a life! Everything was perfect. And I was so happy.

After half a year, he bought us a new house.

I could pick out anything, the furniture, the paint for the walls, the flowers for the garden. He pampered me a lot and kept giving me presents. The biggest gift was a trip to Venice.

And then my sister came to visit. Had I already known what to expect before she arrived, I would have thought twice about leaving them alone in our house. But I was so happy to see her again that I put aside any concerns.

We were sitting at the table when she blurted out the reason for her visit.

"Emma, my husband doesn't like you. You were acting like such a bitch at my birthday party. He was shocked!"

Richard looked at me in surprise and didn't know what to say and then the humiliation came up.

"OUUT! Get out of my house!" I yelled. "Just get the hell out of here. I'm acting like a bitch? Oh really? And what are you doing? Every single time you just walk right into my life and start nagging me. No matter what I achieve in my life, you can't deal with it.

You are the most selfish person I have ever met in my life. Just disappear from my life! And now you come here to humiliate me. I've had enough! Get out of my life."

Richard accompanied her to the door. But instead of having my back and making sure she disappeared as quickly as possible, he quietly whispered to her.

This day was the beginning of the end of my relationship with Richard. It was like poison that spread to me. We argued more and more often.

And my sister was always the reason for the argument. Why didn't I find happiness and peace? I just wanted Richard and me to be happy ...

A few weeks later, she contacted me again. I had troubles dealing with her apology. But at least I wanted to take the time to talk to her.

Richard and I increasingly argued more and more and he became more and more jealous and possessive. Suddenly, I also noticed qualities about him that I had never seen before in him. Did he not love me more? Or was it actually the external circumstances that poisoned our relationship?

I was devastated, it had started so perfectly with us and it all came to an end. And why did my sister always play such a negative role in my relationships?

But apparently that was still not enough to let go. I was shocked, but I loved my sister, too. I longed for harmony in the family and just didn't want to accept that my sister wanted everything for me. She just didn't want me to be happy!

Over time, the distance between Richard and me grew larger and larger. When my sister was visiting, Richard paid a lot of attention to her. And even when she was in Germany, the two wrote themselves unusually often. Did I not see that, or did I perhaps not want to see it?

And then, what I had long been afraid of actually happened. Richard had left for the weekend. With his buddy, or so he said. But when he came back, he was completely changed.

Without warning, he said, "Please move out, Emma. You have one week of time! I'll give you the money for your furniture! Then you can buy new items. Now, I'm gonna live my life, and you can live yours!" He said proudly and hurt at the same time.

I was shocked! "Richard, what happened, is it another woman, you can't just throw me out of the house!" "No, that's not it!" He said ashamed and his glance was stuck to the floor.

What did just happen? Why did the next relationship end now? We were so happy ...

At least I still had my own life. I had kept my beauty salon. My co-workers did a great job and continued to build the studio during my time in Spain.

Besides, I was also a choreographer and dancer. I had my friends and my social life. I suspected that he had just designed his entire life around me. Everything had just been about me. Maybe he loved me more than I loved him? Maybe it was about this little place here. And about Germany.

And what part did my sister have in the break-up of my relationship this time? I decided not to fight it. That would be pointless.

Although I didn't have a flat in Germany anymore, a customer from the beauty salon was a first-class broker. She promised to help me with finding a flat.

I sold the furniture to Richard and made my way to Zurich ....

Vanessa was already waiting for me. What would I expect in Zurich?

A new phase in my life was just about to begin ...

Back to Berlin

... After all this hard time, I decided to leave my old life behind me and to move to Berlin at last. The existing studio continued to run successfully with my 3 employees, which I was very proud of. In the meantime, I lived in a beautiful apartment, big bright rooms turned it into something really special. In the middle of the city, but with a lot of nature around. Just as I had always wished. It was perfect and I planned to open a second beauty salon and had already found competent staff and a suitable space for it.

I also wanted to promote my career as an actress in the big city. I would never give up!

I made a quick decision to sign up for a new workshop and set out on my way there.

I didn't let myself get pushed down by the first workshop and this time I was completely focused. At last, I banished Matthews from my thoughts and so I could fully focus on acting.

But again, I did all honor to my almost unnatural unpunctuality. Completely out of breath, I finally arrived in the big hall of the acting school.

The other participants were already gathered and were waiting for me. This time, there were more participants and a total of four lecturers. The lecturer I had last time was out of sight.

After an extensive round of introductions, each one picked their monologue. And then it really went down to business. Camera acting, dancing, singing.

The choreographer obviously had a bit of a problem with me being a choreographer myself and that I could easily keep up with her. But I didn't let that bother me either.

I also enjoyed the language lessons additionally to the dance performances. We learned to breathe properly and to play with language. It was really great to experience how we could use our voice and what effect we could achieve with the different techniques.

It was just fantastic and exactly what I always wanted to do! And then there was the moment that scared me a little bit. We had to recite our monologues. The point where I failed at the last workshop. "Emma, please come on stage. We are already very excited!"

"That has always been my dream!" I began confidently. "I always wanted to die together with my loved ones. At the same time, so that I don't have to experience, if one dies before the other. Well, I could always have imagined dying with you all .... "

When I finished, I looked around nervously. But this time not only the other participants applauded. The lecturers also seemed enthusiastic. I was really relieved. My whole body was so tense that it almost hurt. But now I felt the sheer relief inside of me.

The very thought of working as an actress motivated me. That has always been my dream. At the age of 14, I dreamed of living in California, L.A one day. I had filled whole albums with my ideas. Cut out and glued in pictures and written small poems.

When the workshop was over, we waited for our individual talk. One after the other, we were called to the lecturers receive the ratings for our monologues.

And this time, what I had hoped for in my dreams happened. "So, dear Emma. I really liked your presentation of the piece. There was something truthful about it. I strongly recommend you to take a private coach. I definitely see you in the movies and not necessarily in the theater! A coach can help you build your skills and deepen what you've learned here."

That was a fantastic feedback. My motivation to work as an actress was finally there!

My second beauty salon went so well that I didn't have to work myself anymore. I was everywhere, at trade fairs, as a make-up artist at weddings, at the theater and - on the set of my first film.

I actually made it and got hold of a small role in a baroque film that took place in the late 16th century. My role was nothing special, a visitor on a ball. A short text. But hey, it was my first role as an actress. It was amazing and exactly what I always wanted.

The experience of being on the other side of the make-up once was incredible. With my eyes closed, I sat there and thoroughly enjoyed being prepared for the role by the make-up artist. My slightly curly hair was pinned up and hidden under a wig. My dress was an ocean blue dream of tulle and lots of fabric. Typical Baroque. The set was crowded, there were people everywhere. Here the camera team, there the extras. In between, the actors whirred around, searching for their seats.

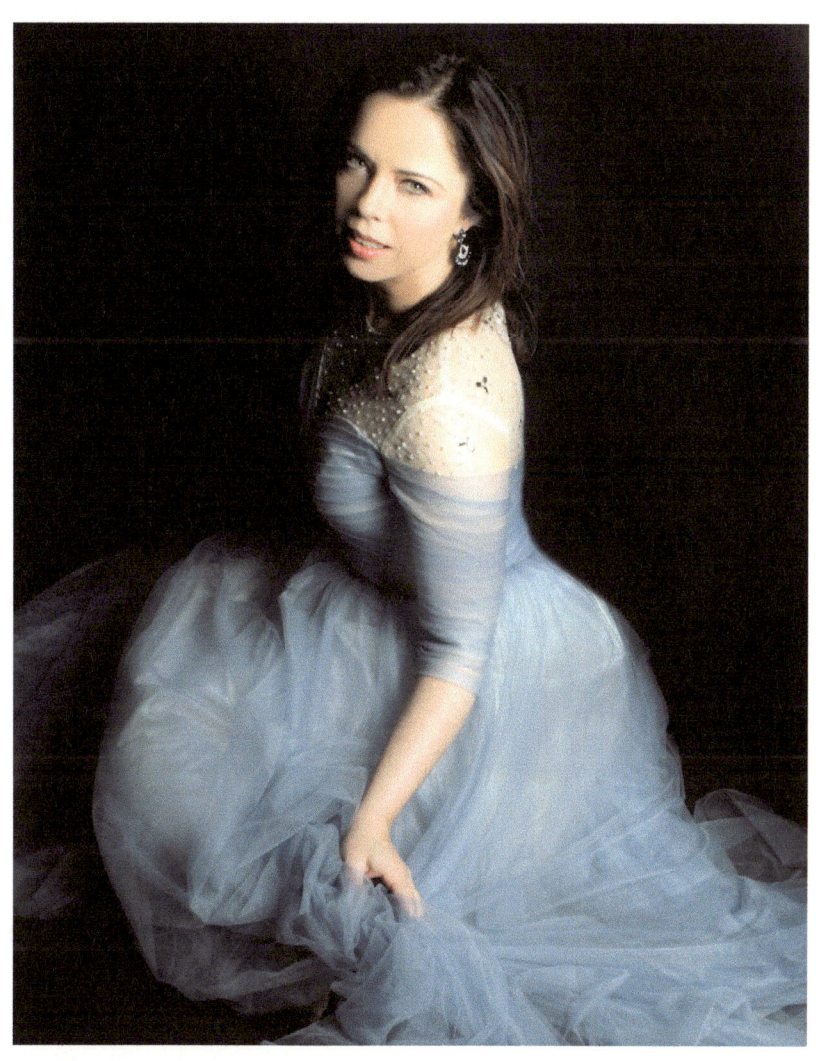

The ballroom was huge. Oversized chandeliers hung from the stucco ceilings, the floor was freshly polished and reflected the chandeliers.

And then it was my turn ...

I was allowed to be on the set for the rest of the week and watch the filming. I wanted more. It was an inspiring, creative profession.

"Hey Emma! Nice to see you!"

I turned and looked straight into the eyes of Ava. "Hey, wow. What are you doing here? I didn't even see you earlier!" I replied joyfully.

"One of the make-up artists couldn't make it, so I jumped in at short notice. And you? You look as if you actually made it, congratulations!"

"Indeed. I've come closer to my goals. And next, we'll implement our plan and make L.A. unsafe!"

Los Angeles II - Reunion with Matthews

Finally, Los Angeles, the city of angels, called for me. It was early in the year when Ava and I flew to Los Angeles. I could already feel the air of the ocean on my skin as we sat in the plane. We would stay with friends from Ava right on the beach in a clubhouse as we had planned.

Since the house belonged to their friends, we could stay there as long as we wanted. We were full of enthusiasm and anticipation. Even the last bit of filming at the set had inspired me so much that now Los Angeles fit perfectly into the plan. I forgot about Matthews. Kind of.......

I still felt the sadness about the loss inside of me. A sadness that overshadowed the anticipation of Los Angeles. "What's up, Emma, what are you thinking about?" Ava asked me. Apparently, Ava knew me better after such a short time than anyone else did! "You know, Ava, I visited somebody in Los Angeles last year and just thought about that time. Matthews is an actor living in Hollywood."

"Ah, those guys! I made some experiences with those myself! Forget about him, we're going to Los Angeles! It's going to be awesome, you'll see!"

I liked her amazing, positive nature and was in a positive mood. I rummaged for a handkerchief in my pocket. But instead, I suddenly held something else in my hand. The USB stick that Zane gave me on my last visit to the United States. We had been in contact all the time and now I had the chance to give the USB stick back to him.

A glance at Ava revealed that she was now asleep. Since it was already late in the evening in German time, I decided to do the same. I closed my eyes and fell asleep right away.

"Ladies and gentlemen, in about half an hour we will arrive in Los Angeles, Please, put your seat into a straight position and put your seatbelts on." The voice of the stewardess woke me up and I immediately felt a tingling sensation in my body. A tingling that I had every time I arrived in this city.

Again, I was dreaming of the long sandy beaches and the fantastic sunsets of Santa Monica ....

"Come on, Emma, stop dreaming, we have to get our bags!" Yes, Ava knew me well. I already appreciated her as a very good friend by my side! After we finally had our luggage and suffered through the customs, we were at the exit of the airport.

There it was again. The incomparable energy of the city. An energy that I didn't feel anywhere else in the world!

It was a mixture of sex, creativity and a dose of marijuana, coupled with passion. A pinch of sun and nature! The perfect mix. Absolutely crazy and dangerous at the same time! What would this city bring me this time …

We didn't have to wait long. Ava's friends were already standing in front of the airport with a black BMW, waiting for us. It was perfect!

"Hey Guys, nice to see you. Ava, honey!" The man hugged Ava tightly. She returned the hug. "Hi, I'm James, and this is my girlfriend, Sienna!"

"Nice to meet you guys, I'm Emma!"

"Really nice to meet you, Emma. Let's go to the clubhouse!"

As soon as we were in the car, the BMW turned into a convertible. The wind made my hair dance and the sun shone right into my face. James turned on his music, it was Chris Brown's "Loyal". I felt LA's sunshine all the way down to my little toe, and I knew what I had missed so much in Germany in the last few months. Here, I felt at home and accepted, here I could be who I was and didn't have to pretend or be liked by anyone superficially. I felt an incomparable sense of freedom.

And then we were there. "Oh my God, that's amazing!" I yelled when I saw the big clubhouse, it was awesome! A whole house for us alone, with a pool and garden, right at the beach! It almost looked like a mansion and was owned by James and Sienna! They were also in the film industry, he was a producer, she was an actress, Ava also worked in productions for a short time and had her own office on the Hollywood Walk of fame. ......

I was so excited! My whole body was throbbing and I can't tell whether it was the tequila James was serving for barbecue, or this wonderful city. I was overjoyed. ... ..

After dinner, Ava suggested driving to Malibu. The drive there was already an experience ....

The wind gently blew into our faces and the sun created a glow on our skin. "Beautiful People" by Chris Brown was playing on the radio.

We were glowing in competition with the sun. On the right side there were mansions, on the left, there was the panorama of the shimmering turquoise blue Pacific Ocean. We let the verses of the song melt in our mouths:

"Live your life, let the love inside, it´s your life the beauty is deep inside inside you, don`t let 'em bring you down...".

Then Ava had the idea to drive to Beverly Hills. There were elegantly dressed people everywhere. From Chanel to Louis Vuitton, everything could be seen. Clothes, handbags, shoes. It was breathtaking. I felt like in an episode of 90210.

Everything was possible. Everything you firmly believe in. This city gives you this energy like no other city.

The Rodeo Drive is considered one of the most expensive shopping streets in the world. I was mesmerized. The shops were of high quality, the sales assistants looked like Jessica Alba. At least that's how it felt to me.

The street where we had lunch was actually Beverly Hills 90210. It was exactly as I had imagined in my childhood dreams. I was in love with California, in love with L.A. The city had taken me in and wouldn't let me go.

Back in the clubhouse, James surprised us with the news that we could go to a private party. He managed to get us onto the guest list there.

I was so excited. A private party, here in L.A., a beach house full of famous people. Or at least those who intended to become famous.

"What should I wear? Ava, I'm so excited. Do you think the blue dress fits the occasion?" I looked at Ava. She looked stunning. Her long, slightly curly hair hung elegantly over her shoulders, along with a wine-red cocktail dress, matching shoes and jewelery! It was a perfect outfit.

"Yes, that fits. Put it on. I would like to see it on you."

Ava thought the dress was good. She chose suitable shoes and lent me a necklace from her valuable collection. "Perfect! Let's go! Let's go drive some men crazy!" We gleefully exchanged meaningful glances and made our way.

The party was just amazing. The location was like a Hollywood block-buster. A huge mansion, all in white. In the garden there was a large pool, and direct private access to the beach.

When we finally made it through the VIP check, we were accompanied through a long corridor by a lady. She showed us and our table and explained where we would find food and drinks.

The guests who joined us at the table were all people from the film and artist industry. I got goose bumps. And then the band started playing. They played rock and pop music and had a perfect choreography. The dancers danced like J Lo, perfectly rehearsed.

I was exactly in the right place at that moment. Here I belonged. Since James and Sienna knew the organizers of this private party, we were allowed to enjoy all that was otherwise reserved for high society. I was in a pink Hollywood bubble that I never wanted to burst.

When the band disappeared from the dance floor, a star DJ took over. The house music he played was awesome.

Ava and I danced wildly and had fun. What a great start. That was the life I wanted to live. I was overjoyed to have followed Ava's invitation and come here with her. We took a break ....

A male voice tore me from my thoughts. I was sitting at the table pondering about my time with Matthews when a hand asked me to dance. When I looked up, a strange man stood in front of me. His six-pack was visible through the shirt, his upper arms looked very muscular. Tanned from the sun, bright short hair. He looked like he came straight from a movie.

"Hi, I`m Bryan. How are you? I would love to dance with you!"

"Hello Bryan, I`m Emma. I`m very well, thank you. Yes, with pleasure!"

Bryan took my hand and pulled me onto the dance floor. I felt like I was on cloud nine. Bryan pulled me closer so I could feel his muscles. We danced for a long time.

"Sorry, I need a break!" I grinned at him. My feet ached from the high heels, but I tried not to show that. Bryan dragged me along and ordered a drink a the bar for me.

As I waited for Brian, a voice that I knew very well spoke to me.

"Emma ..."

When I turned around, I looked deep into his eyes! Matthews! I was speechless ... what was he doing here? That couldn't be true. I was just about to get him out of my head, and then he suddenly stands right in front of me. My facial expression froze. And then I immediately turned red.

I forced myself to stay calm. Just as I was sorting my thoughts to answer, Bryan came back. "Hey Emma, here's your drink!" Bryan handed me my glass and looked from me to Matthews.

Bryan seemed to grasp the situation immediately and stepped subtly into the background. "Matthews, what are you doing ...." I started stuttering, "Emma, let's talk!" Matthews interrupted my attempt to speak. His eyes were sad and demanding at the same time.

"About what? About how you dumped me last year? About how you threw me out of the apartment like it was nothing? Or would you rather talk about the women with whom you had something going on at the same time? Or what exactly do you want to talk about?

Matthews, I really loved you. More than anything else in the world. I was ready to give up everything I had. If you had asked me, I would have stayed with you and would have built up a new life with you here. But what you said was clear enough!"

"Emma, it wasn't like you think. There was nothing going on with Hanna. I love you. That I ditched you like that last year, I am really sorry about. That was the biggest mistake of my life. But I had no choice. Hanna was jealous of you and gave me the choice. You or the apartment. What was I supposed to do. I hardly had any money and couldn't have offered to buy you anything. The jobs I had at the time were badly paid. I..."

"Just drop it! It went the way it did. You can't undo that. My life was a complete mess. It took me several months to recover from you. Now I have managed to build something up. I have achieved my goals. And now I know exactly what I want. And above all, I know what I do not want: YOU!

Get out of my life. I have everything I need. And you certainly are not what I need."

"Let`s go!", I said to Bryan and grabbed his arm. Matthews stayed at the bar with a confused expression on his face. He was still standing at the bar, staring at me like a sheep.

And then she suddenly stood next to him again.

Hanna snuggled up against Matthews and whispered something in his ear. Her eyes went directly to me at the table, it couldn't be any more deceitful and vicious he couldn't be. The two seemed so familiar with each other that I couldn't believe there was one spark of truth in his reason for allowing Hanna to throw me out of the apartment.

A tear ran down my face. I still loved him, no matter how much I wanted to suppress it. But I had made a firm decision. I never wanted to get myself back to the point of losing it.

Never again would I allow a man to treat me like this. These times were finally over.

Bryan was gone too. I was on my way to the bathroom to refresh my makeup when Matthews got in my way. "Emma stop, can we please talk really quickly?" He just wouldn't stop ....

"About what? Everything has been said!" – "No, it hasn't. When I messaged you, suddenly nothing came of you! Why? Emma, I miss you, I love you!"

"Ask Hanna or whoever you're with who answers your messages. Then you know why nothing came from me anymore!"

He looked at me confused again and tried to hold me. "Matthews let me go! I'm going back to my friends now! Take care!" I couldn't believe what I had just said. But right now, it was the only sensible thing I could say.

"Emma!" I heard him calling me, but I didn't look back, Matthew's chapter was finally over.

As the party came to an end, it was time for Ava and me to leave too. On the way to the car I noticed something was wrong

"Emma, everything okay?" Ava asked me.

"Honestly, nothing is ok. That was Matthews, the actor I visited last year. I didn't think meeting him again would bother me like that."

"Emma, if I can do anything for you, let me know. OK?"

"I will do that! For a first, could you please drop me off at the Santa Monica Pier. I'd like to spend some time on my own. I'll walk back to the clubhouse."

Ava drove the car to the side of the road and let me out. "Are you sure? It's the middle of the night!"

"Yes I am. I'll take care of myself. See you tomorrow morning!"

Lost in thought, I walked along the pier. Did I act appropriately? Or should I have given Matthews the opportunity to explain everything to me? And then? He would have probably just kept telling me how sorry he was.

On the other hand, Hanna and he seemed so familiar. Surely, the two were a couple. And then there was the other woman. The one who met him last summer. He sure didn't hesitate when it comes to women.

Apparently, that was already over again. Was he still with Hanna? Why didn't he just move out when he had no feelings for her? Why was he allowing her to blackmail him? Something was going on there. Something forced him to submit to her. I wouldn't know what that was anymore. At least, I didn't want to know anymore.

Arriving at the clubhouse, I took off my shoes and walked barefoot on the warm sand. Nobody was around, I was completely alone. I sat down by the pool and let my feet dangle in the water. The cool water was a blessing to my aching feet.

Then I lied down in one of the sunbeds, looked up at the sky and tried to count the stars.

"Emma, thank God! I've been looking for you everywhere. We were worried." Ava looked at me with a serious expression on her face.

"Did you sleep outside here?"

"Good morning!" I yawned. "Yes, I must have fallen asleep here. Sorry, I didn't mean to scare you."

"Good morning, yeah right. It is 2 o'clock in the afternoon! You over-slept the whole morning. We were about to inform the police! Come on, let's go shopping. I know some really good stores. That will quickly improve your mood I am sure!"

I quickly slipped into the shower and put on comfortable clothes. Jeans, blouse, sneakers. "You really want to go in sneakers?" "Please no high heels, Ava. My feet are still hurting from last night!" We laughed and set off.

And Ava was right. The walk at the Santa Monica Pier was really good. Everywhere you saw artists singing or dancing. The mood was exuberant and let all my worries fade.

I already felt that mood when I was here with Matthews. Matthews, as soon as I thought of him, the tears shot into my eyes. But I had to stay strong. I wanted to stay strong. Matthews definitely didn't do me any good and I was not about to expose myself again to the danger of my life going off track. This chapter should definitely be history.

"Ava, I have some plans. I gotta go." "Do you want to meet Matthews?" She asked me.

"No, Don`t worry. This guy is definitely history. I dumped him.

I met a director in Zurich some time ago. He lives here too. And we decided back then that we would meet for coffee when I'm in L.A. And that's exactly what I want to do now!"

"Aha, you're calling it a coffee!" Ava laughed. Her laughter was so full of life that I let myself be infected.

"Come on, let's go back to the clubhouse. Then you can get ready quickly." Ava and I grabbed our shopping bags and headed off.

I wanted to keep jeans and sneakers on. But Bill had reserved a table in a 5-star restaurant and so I had no choice but to squeeze myself back into elegant clothes. "Oh, what the hell" I thought to myself. After all, I had to get used to this dress style, if I wanted to gain a foothold here in L.A.

At 7 o'clock in the evening, I went to the restaurant. Bill was already there and walked towards me with a huge smile on his face.

"Hi Emma, how long has it been now? I am very glad to see you again!" – "Yes, it has been a long time. But it's really great to see you." With a smile, I linked arms with him.

Our table was on the roof terrace. Just stunning. Slowly, I began to get used to this environment. The pool had a summery atmosphere. We drank martini and ordered something to eat.

"In my feelings" by Drake was playing from the speakers.

"So, Emma ... Tell me about your life. How do you like Los Angeles?"

I was grateful to be distracted and told Bill about the beauty salon that I had opened in Berlin. About my work as a choreographer and dancer. And about the drama workshops. About the fact that I wasn't accepted the first time, he was not surprised. That would happen to many, he reassured me. It is rather abnormal if you do it right off the bat.

He was all the more pleased that the second attempt had gone so well. "Wow! That's sounds great. Did you follow the advice?" He asked me. "Yes, I'm taking some private lessons now. And believe it or not, I already had my first gig in a small movie." I told him proudly.

Secretly, of course, I hoped he would offer me a role in his new horror movie. Who wouldn't be happy about that? That's how many careers start here in Hollywood. But nothing came from him. And I didn't dare ask him. Maybe I wasn't ready yet?

Bill told me that he was very busy these days. The filming of his new film was soon to start and he still had to make some preparations.

"I'm just in love with this city!" I continued. Finally, I felt well again. Finally, I was able to let go and start enjoying my time here in L.A. The moments in which Matthew could make me feel bad with his sudden appearance became fewer and fewer. I was already in the recovery phase again. I was a fighter!

While he told me about the plot of his new movie, he ordered two martinis. The evening was still young.

Slightly drunk, I got out of Bill's car. "Thanks for the evening. It was really great, meeting you again."

"Let's stay in touch, Emma. I'll call you! Enjoy your time in LA."

When I woke up in the morning, the sun was shining straight in my face. It was just 7 o'clock. What an ungodly time. Who got up so early in the morning?

"Emma let's go to Runyan Canyon. Do a little hike. It's not that hot yet." I looked at Ava in disbelief. "It's really nice that you think about me, but this isn't really my time yet." I said to Ava and pulled up my blanket.

"Come on!" Ava pulled the blanket off me again. "Ok, ok. I'm coming already. Give me 5 minutes!" I replied.

In a somewhat revealing sports outfits, we headed out. Our hike took about two hours. Looking down the hills to see Los Angeles almost took my breath away. The view was indescribable.

After that, Ava drove to the Laguna Beach at the Orange County. I used the approximately 1 hour drive to tell Ava about Bill. And then it really came out of me. In the end, Ava knew my whole life story. I told her about Mike, Richard and how I met Matthews at the art exhibition in Zurich. My time in L.A. last summer.

How Hanna threw me out of the apartment and Matthews, who had completely succumbed to her. "Maybe she's his pimp. Who knows!" Ava joked Ava. She made me laugh.

"Sure, and since he didn't want any money from me, she was angry and kicked me out?" – "Something like that!" Ava's laugh was so contagious again that I almost forgot about the world around me.

"Wow, what a dream place!" The view I had was breathtaking. The Laguna Beach had a truly Mediterranean flair, palm trees lined the stairs that went up from the beach to the houses.

By that time, it was 11.30am. We hadn't had breakfast yet and so we decided without further ado to have some extensive breakfast in one of the many cafes.

Later back in the clubhouse, James and Sienna welcomed us in elegant formal wear. "Wow! Where are you planning to go?" Ava asked "Well, we're going to the Grammy after party. You should hurry up. You are both on the guest list, so."

I was completely overjoyed. A Grammy Party! How incredible was that? Quickly, I showered and slipped back into an elegant evening gown. This time I chose the little black one. My wavy hair fell elegantly over my shoulders which worked perfectly with my golden jewelry. That was it. My childhood dream coming true. I actually did it!

The building in which the party was held was barely visible from the outside. We stood in front of an oversized gate and waited to be let in. James spoke through the intercom, the gate opened and we headed straight for the mansion.

I looked around in astonishment. There were cameras everywhere, the security staff was spread all over the grounds. On the parking lots, there was one luxury car next to the other.

Very important persons were attending the party. Otherwise, I couldn't explain what I was seeing. The excitement rose.

The mansion was completely white, just like the one we stayed at the first night. The fronts must have been 70% glass and allowed a lot of light inside. Everything was kept in white and bright colors. There were guests standing around in little groups everywhere. Ava and I went straight to the pool.

I studied the people around me, secretly looking for Matthews. But this time he was nowhere to be seen. Apparently, that was a party he was not invited to. Bad enough that he was already on my mind once again. No matter what I did, he was always present.

"Look!" Ava tore me from my thoughts. My eyes followed her index finger. "Wow, what a view. That's really incredible! A few weeks ago, I was completely devastated and today I am sitting here, in the middle of the hills, at a pool in one of the most beautiful mansions there is, looking directly at the Hollywood Sign."

Ava smiled. "Yes, the sign is also impressive. But that's not what I meant. Look closely. Who's over there on the other side of the pool!"

I squinted. "Pinch me. That can't be true. It looks surreal! The guy looks like Leonardo DiCaprio." He turned and smiled at me.

"Hey, that's Leonardo DiCaprio!"

Ava was just holding me tight. I was so shocked I almost fell into the pool. But just when I was able to gather my courage and go to him, he said goodbye to his friends. And then he was gone.

The party was still an absolute success to me. I managed to talk to a lot of guests. Among them, there were some producers and actors. I exchanged business cards, received invitations and enjoyed the evening to the fullest.

When we all sat together at the breakfast table the next morning, there was much to talk about the evening at the mansion.

James and Sienna listened to me in amusement as I told them I had seen Leo. That was nothing special for the two of them. They lived here, were part of Hollywood and constantly involved with famous actors. But for me it was all like an illusion.

I thought about my family, my friends and my life in Germany. About my tiring, boring everyday life. How much I still loved Matthews and didn't manage to banish him from my thoughts.

But here I was a different person. I was more confident, more creative, stronger and sociable. I felt like I had finally come home.

And then an emptiness overcame me like I'd never seen before. The thought that in 2 days I would fly back to Germany was almost unbearable. What would wait there for me? A beauty salon and an empty, cold apartment. My friends were all around the world. Ava, who often commuted to Berlin, had become a very good friend. But could she fill the void in my heart?

What about love? I missed a man in my life. A person who loved me unconditionally the way I was. With everything I had.

I said goodbye to the others. I wanted to be alone. James lent me his car and so I drove to Runyan Canyon again.

With a water bottle and comfortable sports shoes, I started climbing the mountain. It was pretty steep, but I really wanted to get to the Hollywood Sign. Wanted to clear my mind ....

The heat was almost unbearable, but I fought my way through it. The effort was exactly what I needed now. I felt every muscle in my body, the sweat ran down my forehead. My hair was already wet when I finally arrived on a plateau. Exhausted, I dropped onto the grass.

My eyes went over the area. The view was just fantastic. I was just wondering how far I had to go in order to get to the sign when I saw him.

There he sat. Matthews. I couldn't believe my eyes. He was busy with his cell phone and had headphones on. Had he noticed me? Probably not. Otherwise he would stare at his phone so absent-mindedly.

Just when I decided to go to him, a woman came up to him. She approached Matthews directly, and he turned to hug her. The heartfelt kiss between the two broke my heart ....

But maybe that was exactly what I needed to understand who Matthews really was.

A pretty boy who shuffled from woman to woman and could never manage to stay with one permanently. Someone who used women and always looked for someone to take care of him. Presumably, this was the next rich woman he could use.

My heart was finally broken. Intuitively I wanted to go further to the sign. Far up, far enough to fall so low that nothing and nobody could save me.

My steps became faster and faster. I ran up the mountain. Past the Hollywood Sign until I came back up a hill. And there I sat now. Totally out of breath. Every muscle ached - and so did my torn heart. There's a difference in imagining something – and then actually seeing it happen: Matthews with another woman.

Unhindered, I let my feelings run free. I screamed, I cried, I punched the ground.

WHY? Why did this just happen to me?

I had everything! I was lying on the grass, in the sunset. Below me, there was the Hollywood Sign. Everything I had ever dreamed of was within reach. I knew at least a dozen producers, had several contacts in the movie industry of Hollywood.

But Matthews was just too present. I didn't manage to banish him from my thoughts, from my heart.

Nothing could calm me down. The great friends that I had found, the fact that I had seen Leonardo DiCaprio in person, that I was in this great city, that I had achieved so much in my life that I was almost at the end of my dreams.

Nothing comforted me anymore. The love I felt for this person was completely broken. What did I expect? Didn't I have eyes in my head? Was I so blind last summer that I didn't realize what was going on?

Wasn't it obvious? When Hanna threw me out of the apartment? What did he want to tell me that night at the club? I just stared into the sky above me. It hurt so much. I couldn't imagine that anyone on this earth had ever felt such pain as I felt right now.

Why did I always have to experience this suffering? Would I ever find my happiness? Or was I destined to search for my soulmate forever? I thought I found my soulmate in Matthews.

But he had lied to me, betrayed me and deceived me. He probably had something going on with Hanna or another woman, and I was with him all the time, serving as a means to an end. Tears ran down my cheeks. I felt humiliated, ashamed, exploited. What should I do now?

My mobile buzzed. It showed 10 missed calls and 3 messages. It was Ava who was worried. "Hey Chica, where are you? Please call me back, we are very worried!"

I put my phone next to me. I just couldn't answer. Should I go back? Could I ever go back? Did I still have a life worth living for? I looked around. Slowly I walked to the cliff that was just in front of me. Should I close my eyes and just let myself be surprised if I no longer had ground under my feet? Or head for the end with open eyes? I felt a pressure on my chest like never before!

Was that the problem? Have I never really overcome my difficult childhood and adolescence? Did I fail privately by not allowing myself to feel happy? Couldn't I confess that I deserved happiness? Which one was it? What was the reason that I was not really happy? I didn't know it. Thousands of thoughts ran through my mind at once. A pure rollercoaster of thoughts.

As I stood on the precipice, I reviewed my life. My childhood, which was happy and beautiful in Russia. My childhood and youth in Germany, which was terrible. My family, my love affairs, my friendships. The many trips to all the countries, my career, my successful studio, the first film role, the passionate and intense nights with Matthews, the love for him, the years of friendship with Vanessa, the new friendship with Ava, Los Angeles, "the city of angels" ...

My life ran before my eyes in pictures. Maybe that's how you feel and see your life when you're sensing its end ...

The pictures after the truck accident were the same.

The accident, on my sister's birthday. Should I have been dead by now?

Suddenly, I thought of Peg Entwistle, a US actress who in 1932 jumped to her death from the letter H of the world-famous Hollywood sign. Unfortunately, she became known only after her death. That's probably the dark side of Hollywood ....

I looked down and was scared. Should I really jump? What would I leave behind? What was I supposed to think about so shortly before my death? My dark side was completely controlling me. I was ready to put an end to everything. Here and now - I just couldn't do it anymore. Just two more steps ....

...No!!!! I didn't do it, I wanted to live. And then everything turned black around me.

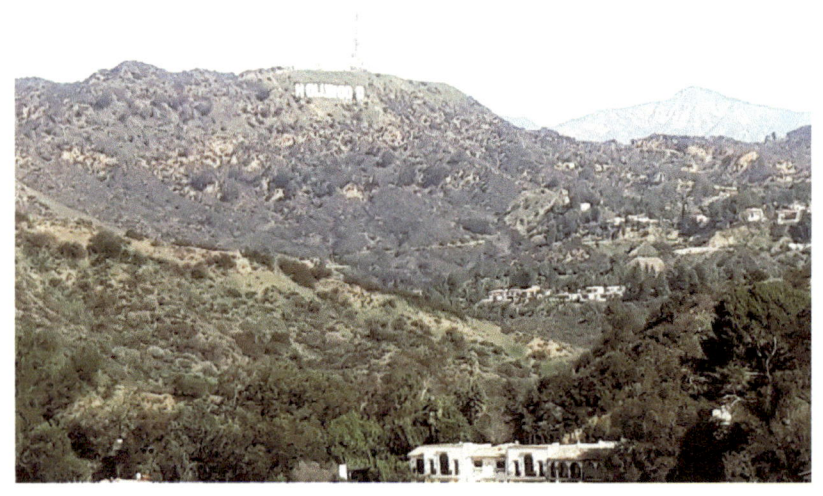

Flight or destination?

I've spent days lying in my bed in the clubhouse. I only told my friends the bare essentials! Of course, I didn't tell them that I almost jumped off the cliff of the Hollywood Signs. But they realized that I wasn't feeling well. They didn't ask why and lovingly cared for me. Ava canceled our flights and stayed with me. She didn't want to leave me like that, but also felt that I was not able to fly back to Germany.

I insisted that the room stayed dark and I didn't allow anyone but Ava, James and Sienna close to me.

Most of the time I just slept. In between, Ava made sure I got fluids into my body.

Slowly but surely, with the help of my friends, I got new courage to live again. My walks on the beach got longer every day, my mood brightened.

And then, after what felt like an eternity, I finally broke my silence. Ava and I sat on the beach and watched the waves. Unexpectedly, I began to speak, and didn't stop until I had talked all my sorrows of my soul.

Ava was sitting next to me all the time listening to me patiently. "You know, Emma, life is not always easy. Probably everyone has met stupid people who are trying to stop them and keep them small. Here in Hollywood too, life is not always pure sunshine. Again, it is raining, people are coming into your life and they are leaving. Sometimes quiet, sometimes with a bang. You will experience the same over here and in Germany. Or in any other country. After all, it doesn't matter where you are. Or where your friends are.

You are a wonderful woman! You have achieved a lot in your life. Two beauty salons, both doing so well that you can easily be away for several months. You are a great choreographer and dancer and have a lot of fun as a make-up artist. Don't let yourself be disturbed by men like Matthews. Such guys aren't worth you ruining your life over them."

I leaned against Ava's shoulder. The calmness that radiated from her slowly transferred to me. I calmed down and started to see light again.

That evening, for the first time since my collapse, I sat down with the others at the table. I didn't want to leave yet, I didn't have the strength to do that yet. Too big was the fear of meeting Matthews and breaking down again.

"Ava, I decided to stay here for a while. I don't know yet how exactly I am going to do that because we've been here for 11 weeks, but I'll find a way.

I don't know yet how I'll react when I meet Matthews, but I don't want to go back to Germany yet."

"You can stay as long as you want, Emma. We have enough space here in this house. And so I can help you get a visa. I may talk to the leading makeup artist at my set. Our next movie is getting about to be filmed. She probably needs one more make-up artist."

James immediately got up and started phoning. Did I just dream that? Did James really just offer me to work as a make-up artist in Hollywood?

Ava smiled meaningfully. "And I have my studio here, too. There is also work for you. And who knows, maybe you will play a role in a movie here, too. But I have to go back to Berlin soon. I am needed there for a major contract."

When we arrived at the airport, I hugged Ava again. "Thank you so much for everything. You literally saved my life!" "See you! I'll be back soon!", Ava replied and disappeared at the terminal.

Sad as I was, I went back to the car. I would miss Ava so much.

A few weeks passed. I got several jobs through my friends and contacts here, which I did passionately.

I went to the Hollywood Sign and walked up to the place where I wanted to end my life. I looked into the deep abyss and got goose bumps all over my body. How could I only think of something like that? But I put aside my recurring negative thoughts and listened to Ava. I stayed strong and became even stronger as a person! I wouldn't end my life for anyone, no matter how painful ....

I also prepared for my next meeting with Bill. He had contacted me on a very nice day when I drove to the clubhouse in Venice Beach saying:

"Hello Emma I thought about giving you a role in my movie. The filming days are going to start the next days. There you're going to learn everything else. I'm gonna send you the script already. The filming begins in Paris and ends in Los Angeles. Best, Bill"

I immediately agreed and couldn't believe it. Finally, a huge grin was on my face. I was so happy to fly to Paris.

All the dreams I had painted in my little book as a child on the floor became true; a little collage of a horror movie as a title - with me as an actress in it.

Amazing, right? I think that's the law of positive attraction. That's the positive power that I'm talking about. You should always be careful what you wish for, because it may come true.

Dreams can come true - just believe, visualize and never lose hope in life!

As Walt Disney said:

"If you can dream it, you can do it!"

Eventually, the pain and the effort will reward you. And now the day had come when the wishes of my childhood dreams became reality.

I didn't hesitate a minute and packed my suitcase in anticipation for the filming days in Paris. This city, too, probably attracted me and my life in a magical way.

Forgotten was all my suffering and the pain of childhood and adolescence ... the critical and devastating words, my anxious overprotective mother, my sister who did was good to me and somehow conjured something evil at the same time, all the wrong friends and relationships.

Matthews was probably only a key figure of my life - one that might just come into my life to open my way as an actress ...

"Oh Chica, I will miss you, off you go to Paris, to the city of love, with the role of your life! You are always welcome here, you know that, right?" ... The smile on Ava's face was as bright as the sun.

"Ava, see you soon!" I laughed determined.

All three of them accompanied me to the airport. Ava was back in LA and wanted to say goodbye to me along with my hosts. I couldn't suppress my tears.

These people had saved me, touched my soul and were always there for me - each one for themselves and together - even in bad times. This is rare.

We hugged each other one last time. I ran to the terminal with a laughing and a crying tear on my face.

Finally, on the airplane, I took a deep breath. On this flight I had enough time to further learn my script for my role in Paris. Ava had downloaded really good music on my I-pad.

I looked at the passing clouds from the airplane window and finally felt free. I could finally take a deep breath after a long time. It cost me all my strength but at last, I was ready to embark on the role of my new life, which was now waiting for me in Paris.

Joyfully, I let my fingers move through the pages of the script. That was a lot of text this time. But I could do it - thanks to Bill. I had my strength back. Incidentally, the script was great, with interesting changes and characters in it ... I slowly came to the last pages.

In 2 hours, we were supposed to land.

Curiously, my fingers brushed through the last pages; the attachment with the actor overview was on the last page. I felt panic rising inside of me. Matthews ... he was on the list!

Was he on the same plane? My blood froze in my veins, the beautiful music fell silent around me and I started feeling nauseous and dizzy.

Terrified, I pushed myself deeper and deeper into the seat; this fear I hadn't felt for such a long time suddenly came creeping up on me again.

The next 2 hours should be the worst of my life so far. Matthews was on board, I sensed that.

To be Continued ....